THE
You Can Do It!
KIDS DIET™

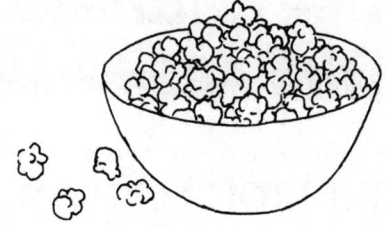

Dee Matthews
with Allan Zullo and Bruce Nash

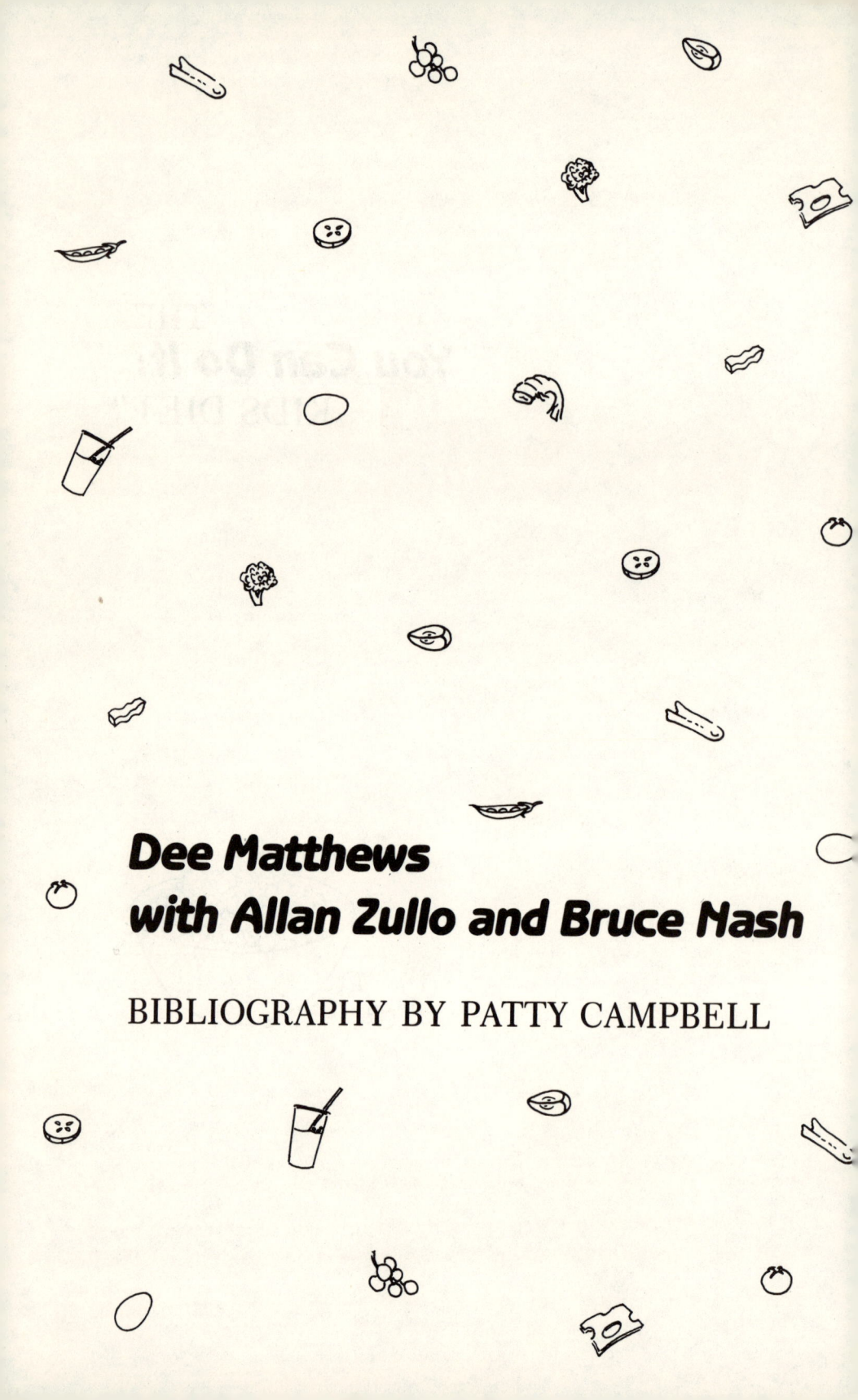

BIBLIOGRAPHY BY PATTY CAMPBELL

THE You Can Do It! KIDS DIET™

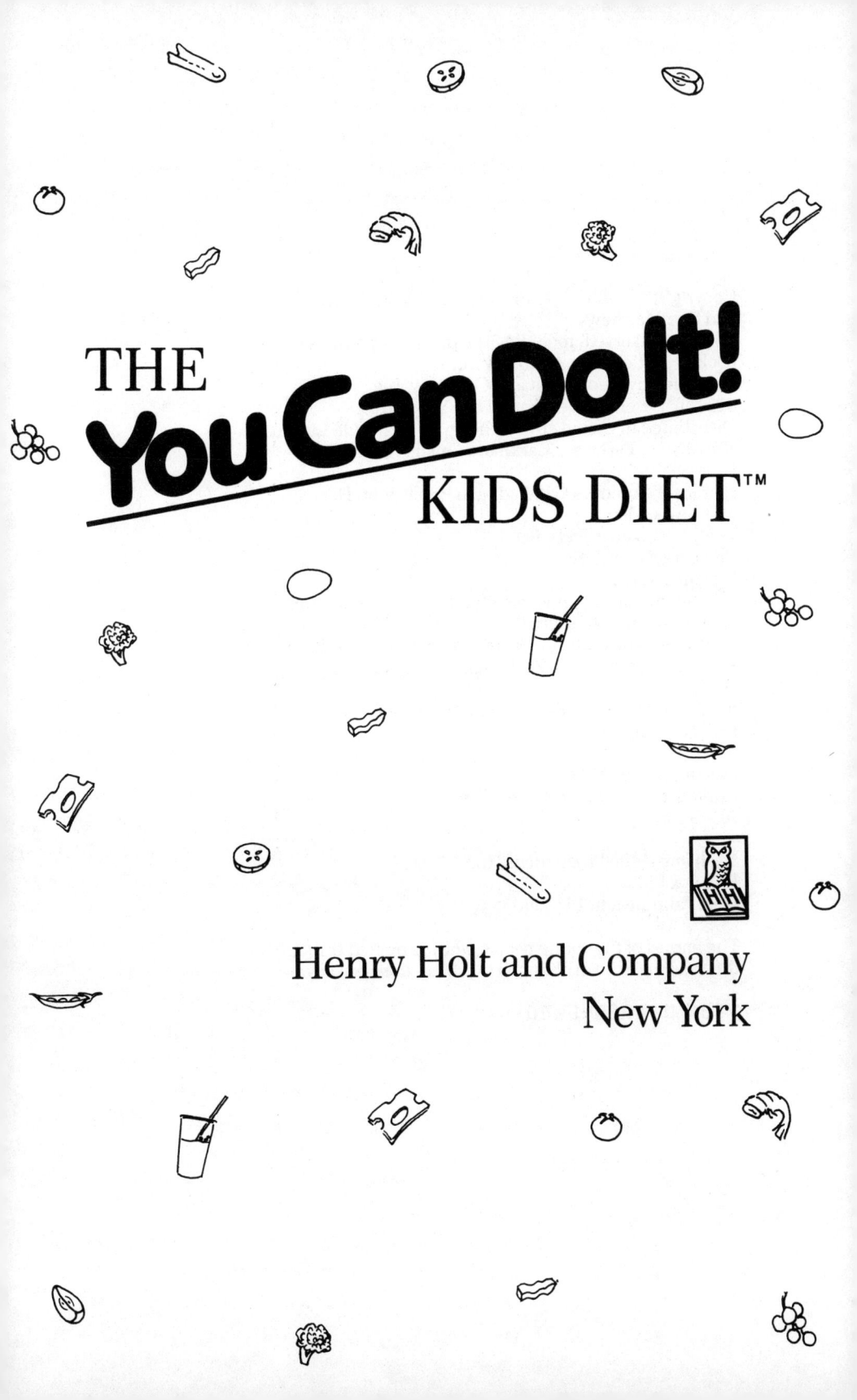

Henry Holt and Company
New York

Copyright © 1985 by Nash and Zullo Productions, Inc.,
and Dee Matthews
All rights reserved, including the right to reproduce this
book or portions thereof in any form.
Published by Henry Holt and Company, Inc.,
521 Fifth Avenue, New York, New York 10175.
Distributed in Canada by Fitzhenry & Whiteside Limited,
195 Allstate Parkway, Markham, Ontario L3R 4T8.

Library of Congress Cataloging in Publication Data
Matthews, Dee.
The you can do it! kids diet.™
Bibliography: p. 241
Includes index.
1. Reducing diets—Juvenile literature.   2. Reducing diets—Recipes—Juvenile literature.   3. Children—Nutrition—Juvenile literature.   4. Obesity in children—Juvenile literature.   I. Zullo, Allan.   II. Nash, Bruce.   III. Title.
RM222.2.M378   1984   613.2'5   84-8944
ISBN 0-8050-0620-6

Design by Amy Hill
Printed in the United States of America
10 9 8 7 6 5 4 3 2

Nash and Zullo Productions, Inc.
P.O. Box 6218
West Palm Beach, FL 33405

The names of the young people who are quoted throughout this book have been changed to protect their privacy.

ISBN 0-8050-0620-6

*To you, the reader,
for having the determination
to improve your life.*

Acknowledgments

We wish to thank all the young people in the Diet Encounter program and their parents, who openly and willingly shared with us their thoughts and experiences. We also extend our gratitude to the doctors, registered dietitians, nutritionists, and other health care professionals who gave us valuable advice and suggestions. And most important, we thank our spouses John, Kathy, and Sophie for encouraging and assisting us throughout this endeavor.

—D.M., A.Z., B.N.

Contents

FOREWORD *xi*
HOW TO USE THIS BOOK *xiii*

You Can Do It! *1*

GROWING UP FAT 5

1 My Battle with Fat *7*
2 Fat Isn't Fun *19*
3 Why You Are Fat *29*

GOING ON THE DIET 47

4 Making Up Your Mind *49*
5 Get Ready, Get Set . . . *55*
6 The Diet *67*

7 Fourteen-Day Sample Menu *81*
8 Taking Charge *98*
9 Recipes *107*
10 The Good Eating Habit *123*
11 The First Two Weeks *128*
12 The Rest of the Way *136*

COPING ON THE DIET *141*

13 Coping with Temptation *143*
14 Coping in School *151*
15 Coping on Holidays and at Special Events *160*
16 Coping at Parties *166*
17 Coping in Restaurants *171*
18 Coping on Vacations and at Summer Camp *175*
19 Coping at Home *182*
20 Oops! *194*

REACHING YOUR GOAL AND STAYING THERE *199*

21 The Big Moment *201*
22 Maintaining Your Ideal Weight *208*
23 Seven-Day Sample Maintenance Menu *217*
24 A Slim New Life *225*

DEAR PARENT . . . *230*
SOME OTHER BOOKS YOU'LL WANT TO READ *241*
INDEX *247*

Foreword

As a pediatrician, I treat many young people of different ages. I'm used to helping kids with many of their problems in growing up.

One of the biggest problems that many of my patients face is being overweight. Somehow it seems to creep up on them, and before they or their parents or their doctors know it, they are just plain too fat.

Being a teenager is full of enough challenges without having to handle the additional burden of a weight problem. Fat is no fun. Some studies show that overweight young people are discriminated against in school and in jobs. For example, even though a fat teenager may be best for a particular job, someone else who is thinner may get the job instead. This seems unfair, but unfortunately it is a fact of life. Also, teenagers who weigh too much can develop serious medical problems such as diabetes, high blood pressure, heart and lung disease, and ailments of the joints. This is especially sad since these problems can often be prevented by simply losing weight.

But losing weight is not easy for young people (or adults, for that matter). You need to follow a sensible, safe, effective diet. Just as important, you need motivation. You must want to do whatever it takes to slim down.

Motivating young people to lose weight and take better care of themselves is where Dee Matthews really excels. She herself has felt the pain and suffering of growing up fat, so she easily relates to young people and their weight problems. As founder of a weight-loss program called Diet Encounter in Palm Beach County, Florida, Dee has helped thousands of young people live slim new lives. I have sent many of my overweight patients to Diet Encounter classes. These young people have returned to my office later with positive attitudes, glowing faces, and trimmer bodies. They are justifiably proud of themselves and have acquired a whole new outlook on life.

They are no different from you except that they have attended Diet Encounter classes. Although you may not have the opportunity to attend such classes, this book will make it seem as though you are sitting right in the front row listening to Dee's advice and hearing the comments of dieting young people. That's what makes this diet book so different from all others. I've seen what this diet can do for my patients. Imagine what it can do for you.

—Elizabeth Brown, M.D., Pediatrician
North Palm Beach Children's Clinic
Palm Beach Gardens, Florida

How to Use This Book

Please read this book through once carefully so you can grasp the basics of the diet. When you are actually following the diet, refer to the chapters that deal with your particular situation, such as how to handle the first two weeks, how to cope with teasing at school, or what to do when you fall off the diet for a day or two.

Although this book is aimed at those young people with a serious weight problem, almost every suggestion and guideline in the following pages can apply to any young person who needs to lose weight—whether it is ten pounds or one hundred pounds.

Before going on this or any diet, obtain the approval of your doctor. Once you begin dieting, make sure you visit your doctor periodically or, at the very least, keep him or her fully informed of your progress.

THE
You Can Do It!
KIDS DIET™

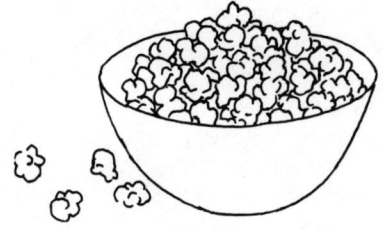

You Can Do It!

You can solve your weight problem once and for all.

That's right, YOU. Not me, not your parents, not your doctor.

Really, it's all up to you.

There are no secrets, no nifty tricks to losing weight. It's all pretty basic stuff. You must eat less and eat better foods. You must be physically active. And you must make a commitment to diet, put forth a strong effort, shoulder the responsibility, and display plenty of determination. I can't do any of those things for you. But what I can do in this book is show you how to

- ✔ Slim down to the weight that is ideal for you
- ✔ Maintain your ideal weight
- ✔ Break bad eating habits and develop good ones
- ✔ Cope with the diet in everyday life, such as at home, at school, on vacation, at parties, and on holidays

I won't dazzle you with fancy tips and clever recipes. I won't give you some magic formula that guarantees dieting will be a breeze.

Instead, this book will provide you with a basic approach, a no-nonsense method that puts you in total control of your own diet. If you are old enough to read this book, then you are old enough to take responsibility for your body, your health, and your well-being. On the You Can Do It! Kids Diet, you are in control of what you eat, how you eat, the way you eat, as well as the amount and kind of physical activity you wish to do.

It's a simple diet that averages between 1,400 and 1,500 calories a day. Don't worry, you don't have to count calories as long as you follow the diet closely. (Many people are no good at counting calories—and they have the figures to prove it.) You won't go hungry. Each day you eat three filling meals plus an after-dinner snack that provide you with proper nutrients, including the necessary vitamins and minerals. The foods are standard fare found in any grocery store—nothing strange or exotic.

You're probably dying to know what's on the diet, right? The first thing most diet book readers do is flip through the pages to see what they can eat on the diet. So go ahead and turn to pages 67–74 and look over the heart of the diet.

You are probably wondering how much weight you can lose each week. You will shed from five to eight pounds the first week and about an average of two pounds each week after that. Losing any faster than that could mean serious health problems. Let's face it, you didn't get fat overnight and you can't expect to lose it all so fast either. It's going to take time. By losing weight gradually and safely, you should never have to diet again. If you don't do something now, you will stay fat (or get even fatter).

Notice I use the word "fat." Don't be offended. It's a word I use often because it's much better than saying such words as *obese, husky, plump, fleshy, portly, tubby, chubby, rotund, beefy, heavyset,* or *pudgy.* We're dealing with fat. We're trying to get rid of it. There is no pussyfooting around with this problem. It's too serious. That's why this book is all straight talk.

It breaks my heart to see so many fat young people. Tomorrow when you go to school, take a close look at your fellow students. You will notice that about one out of every four is overweight (weighing at least 20 percent more than they should for their age, height, and sex). You are one of the more than 20 million American kids who are overweight.

You are also one who can lose weight—if you are determined to work hard at dieting. Ever since this diet was developed in South Florida, it has helped more than two thousand young people like you—even those who had tried and failed on other diets. The success rate of those who have reached their weight goal and maintained control of their weight for a year or longer is 84 percent. I promise that if you follow the guidelines in this book, you will reach your ideal weight too.

Imagine, in just a matter of months, you won't be fat anymore. You will be starting a whole new life as a happy, proud, confident, *slim*, young person. Best of all, you will feel that since you succeeded in reaching such a difficult goal you can accomplish almost anything else you have in mind.

Sound good to you? Then tell yourself, *You Can Do It!*

Growing Up Fat

1

MY BATTLE WITH FAT

I understand how you feel about your weight problem and I know what you are going through. You see, I was a fat kid.

My whole life revolved around food. No matter what I was doing, I was always stuffing my face. I binged on buttered popcorn and candy at the movies, turned slumber parties into night-long refrigerator raids, and went to birthday parties dying to load up on cake and ice cream.

It didn't take a genius to figure out why I was fat. I ate all the time. I think my friends were convinced that eating made me hungry.

I didn't really blimp out until the summer before seventh grade. Somehow the foods at the beach concession stands, at the park picnics, and on family vacations were just too tempting to resist. By the end of June, I heard comments like, "You're adding a little weight, aren't you?" I didn't pay any attention to them. A month later, relatives said, "You seem to be getting awfully chubby." Again, I ignored the remarks. By the end of August, I was told, "Boy, are you fat!" They were right. I had gained a whopping 30 pounds over the summer.

I entered seventh grade standing 4 feet, 10 inches tall and weighing a hefty 135 pounds. I was made painfully aware of how fat I was when all the students were weighed by the school nurse. After I stepped on the scale, the nurse said in a voice loud enough for everyone to hear, "My, my. Someone needs to go on a diet." Talk about embarrassment. I ran into the girls' bathroom, wishing there was a button to push so I could disappear. Did the incident spur me to diet? Nope. I continued to eat my way to "fat city" over the next two years. The only thing bigger than my appetite was my stomach. By ninth grade I stood 5 feet 8 inches and tipped the scale at a gross 225 pounds. That was 85 pounds overweight.

Those years in school as a fatso were the worst of my life. Students poked fun at me: "Where'd you get that dress? From Omar the tentmaker?" "Could you please move? You're blocking out the sun." Those comments were cruel . . . and they certainly hurt.

I'll never forget the time in social studies when the teacher pointed to a map of one of the Great Lakes, referring to it as "a big body of water," and the class clown blurted out, "Wow, that looks just like Dee's figure." The whole class roared. I wanted to drown him.

By far the most humiliating moments for me in school occurred in gym class. I dreaded P.E. more than anything else in the world. I came in last in every race. Nobody wanted to pick me for a team unless it was as the backstop in a softball game. I hated the rope climb most of all. Since I didn't ever want to play Tarzan's Jane, and I never expected to swing across a river, I tried to convince the gym teacher that doing the rope climb was pointless. But she insisted that I do it in order to pass the class. There were five of us fatties who had trouble climbing the stairs, let alone the rope. I tried and I tried but my arms couldn't hoist my overweight body. To this day I can still hear the snickers from my classmates when the teacher ordered four students to get underneath me and lift me up to help get me started. It was like trying to shove a hippo up a willow tree.

Naturally, I wore the largest gym suit you could buy. (It had to be specially ordered because no store carried one in my size.) Once I had struggled into the one-piece outfit, I was okay—until I tried to get out of it. Usually we five fatties had to help each other "peel out," only to face the most horrible part of gym class—the showers.

I always tried to wait until the other students were finished before I showered, so they wouldn't see me naked. I was too ashamed of my rolls of fat. Forget modesty. I was given a towel that was so small it barely dried my hands. Trying to wrap it around my body was like trying to cover a cement truck with a handkerchief. After I patted my face and arms, the towel was dripping wet and I still had an awful lot more body to dry. With the bell about to ring, I fought to get my too-tight clothes on my still-damp body. More often than not, I ended up late for my next class.

I couldn't take the embarrassment anymore. In desperation, I lied to my doctor, saying my bronchitis acted up whenever I attended gym class, so he wrote a note that excused me from further P.E.

As a fat student, I didn't look for attention because I didn't like myself or the way I looked. I didn't join in any extracurricular activities or make many friends. I wanted to do things but I lacked self-confidence. I was afraid to run for student council, to audition for the school play, to join a social club.

I didn't participate much during class. I sat in the back of the classroom so no one would have to look at me and wonder about the size of my wide hips, big belly, and fat arms. Once in shorthand class, the teacher told me to stand up and she proceeded to tell everyone that I had scored the highest grade on a test. Most kids would have felt proud. I felt flustered, praying the teacher would shut up so I could sit down and never be seen again.

Despite the incident, I continued to study hard in all

subjects to earn top grades. When I made straight A's, some students acted as if they wanted to be my friends. I remember once on a Monday night, a popular girl named Sally called me for the first time and invited me to go bowling with her Saturday afternoon. That sounded like a great idea. I was thrilled to think Sally wanted to begin a friendship with a "lardo" like me. On Wednesday Sally stopped me in the hall and asked, "Dee, can you help me out? I was so busy working on the homecoming float last night that I didn't get a chance to do that science report. Could you let me look at yours?" I knew this was cheating but I wanted to be her new friend so much that I gave her my report to copy. On Friday, when I asked Sally what time we would meet at the bowling alley, she said, "Oh, Dee, I'm so sorry. I forgot to tell you that my parents and I are going to my grandparents' house this weekend. We'll have to go bowling another day." Of course, "another day" never came.

This type of trick was pulled on me many times by several students. As soon as they got what they wanted from me, they wouldn't talk to me again until they needed my help with another assignment. Although deep down inside I knew they were just using me, I continued to let them take advantage because for a few brief moments I let myself feel accepted.

I was hardly a social butterfly. On weekends, while other girls went on dates, I stayed home or baby-sat or gossiped on the telephone with my fat girlfriends. We tended to stick together for support and often gathered in my kitchen to make fudge—which we ate as fast as we could make it. Between bites we talked about the boys we wished would ask us out, knowing full well there was little chance they would call us for a date.

That was never made more clear to me than the day Derek, a guy known for his brutal honesty, admitted to me that he was afraid to take me out because he didn't want his buddies to tease him about dating a fat girl like me. He told me point blank, "If you weren't so overweight, I'd ask you out for a date." I stood there and didn't say a word. I was angry. Not at him but at myself. I wanted to go out with him and I knew that the only thing standing between us was my blubber. Unfortunately, I was still not ready to diet. When I got home from school that day I was so upset with myself that I polished off half an apple pie.

Mondays were extra hard on me because that's when the slender girls told me all about the wonderful times they had had over the weekend with their boyfriends. There wasn't much for me to contribute to the conversation other than to describe the TV shows I had watched on Saturday night.

I envied the girls not only for all the fun they had but also for all the neat clothes they wore. Whenever I walked into a store, the salesclerk sent me to the back where the fat girls' clothes—all four different styles—were hanging on racks. If I headed for the dressing room with a few clothes draped over my arm, the saleslady scurried in right behind me with a worried look in her eyes, as if I were a wild gorilla ready to rip her merchandise apart. Actually, she had reason to worry. I grunted and groaned, huffed and puffed as I tried to wriggle into a dress two sizes too small. Usually when I walked out of the dressing room, I left behind popped buttons, broken zippers, and split seams. This was followed by a stern lecture from my mother: "Well, don't expect to go shopping anymore unless you start losing weight." It reached the point where we made two trips a year for clothes—to a big-ladies' store.

I always felt self-conscious at family get-togethers, reunions, and weddings. I tried every excuse in the book not to go to these family functions because I knew I faced an onslaught of comments about my weight. One of my uncles always pinched my cheeks, patted my tummy, and said, "Gee, everybody grew so tall. What happened to you? You grew sideways." Everybody laughed at me. I fumed and pouted. "Your uncle didn't mean to hurt you," my aunt told me. "He was just having a little fun. It's okay." I wasn't okay. His put-downs hurt more than if they had come from a complete stranger.

There was only one consolation in my life—food. And lots of it. After school I often stopped at the neighborhood grocery store and bought four candy bars. I ate two of them on the way home and hid the rest in my bedroom to munch on before dinner. Food helped me cope with my problems. When I fought with a friend or nearly flunked a pop quiz or was zinged by a cruel fat joke, I sought comfort in glazed doughnuts or a pint of ice cream. On the other hand, when I aced a mid-term exam or received a rare compliment from a friend, then I celebrated with some fattening baked treat.

Supper was the day's highlight for me. Every night in our household of eight, the dinner table sagged under enough platters, bowls, and dishes of food to feed the high school marching band. When it came to eating, I played a mean knife and fork—with encores.

Every once in a while, after a long hard look in the mirror, I would attempt a new diet. Once I ate nothing but apples for three days until I couldn't stand to look at applesauce, apple juice, or even apple pie. For the next six months, I wanted to throw up every time I spotted an apple tree. I tried powdered diet drinks to curb my appetite but they tasted like ground-up wet cardboard. As a result, I ate everything in sight to get rid of the awful taste that lingered in my mouth. At other times I tried a liquid diet, a lettuce diet, a vegetable diet, and every other fad diet. But all they did was give me an upset stomach and cramps.

When I entered my junior year in high school, I had the physique of a defensive lineman—5 feet, 8 inches tall, 265 pounds, 40 pounds more than when I started high school. I was depressed. After school, I spent hours in my room listening to music, eating candy bars, and feeling sorry for myself. I let my appearance go down the drain until I looked more like a bag lady than a teenager. I didn't care what I wore, whether I mixed polka dots with stripes or red with orange. I didn't brush my hair. I would face the mirror and shout, "I'm fat, horrible, and disgusting! Why bother putting on makeup or fixing my hair? I'm ugly anyway. No sense using perfume because who's going to say I smell nice?" I hated myself and what I had become.

But then one day as I began to bawl myself out in the mirror once again, I burst into tears. "I'm tired of being fat, tired of being teased, tired of missing out on life." I yearned to have fun like everyone else. I wanted to have boyfriends and go for rides in convertibles and take romantic barefoot walks on the beach. I wanted to make new friends and play basketball and learn ballet and do hundreds of other things. I knew the first step toward those goals was to lose weight. I made up my mind to stick to a rigid diet. But almost immediately I was filled with self-doubts. Could I really succeed? Could I lose all that weight? Did I have enough determination?

My mother was very supportive and took me to the doctor for an examination. Unfortunately, the doctor was unbelievably insensitive to my problem. After pronouncing me a physical wreck, he told my mother, "Forget a diet. Dee is beyond help. She'll die before she's twenty-one." My mind whirled with fear and anger. As I left his office I cried and cursed the doctor with every breath. I vowed on the spot that no matter how long it took, or how hard it would be, I was going to lose all the weight necessary to fit into a size 10 dress. That meant dropping down sixteen sizes and shedding 125 pounds. Nothing was going to stop me from succeeding. I conjured up a mental picture of what I wanted to look like when I reached my goal: an upper body that tapered to a thin waist, rounded hips, and long, slender legs.

I asked for help from no one. This was something I had

to do by myself, for myself. Since there was no diet for young people back then, I read everything I could about proper nutrition and then made up my own diet. (Based on what I know today, that old diet was not safe, so please don't try it.) For breakfast I had a hard-boiled egg and grapefruit juice. Lunch consisted of a piece of lean meat, a vegetable, and a small salad. I ate nothing for dinner except coffee or tea. For weeks my stomach growled and grumbled in protest. I suffered headaches and cramps in my legs.

But nothing—not even my grandparents' concern that I was needlessly harming myself—could deter me from my goal. Although my parents worried about me, they supported my effort.

I began my diet in January of my junior year and by the start of summer vacation, I had dropped nearly 80 pounds. Throughout the summer, I lived like a hermit, avoiding friends, not going to the beach, and not even attending Mass on Sunday. I deliberately became a shut-in because I wanted to wait until I reached my goal before making a grand entrance as the new me, much like the ugly caterpillar that suddenly emerges as a beautiful butterfly. I couldn't wait for the day when I could slip into a size 10. Until then, I refused to buy any new clothes, deciding instead to use safety pins, belts, and ropes to take in my oversized blouses and skirts. What a sight! My clothes were getting so big on me that I looked like a circus clown. But I didn't care. I was averaging a weight loss of 15 pounds a month and I was coming ever so close to my goal.

What a glorious day it was when I stepped on the scale and the needle stopped at 140 pounds. I let out a shriek of joy. "I did it! I did it!" I shouted. In eight tough months I had dropped 125 pounds. Now it was time to celebrate by buying a whole new wardrobe just in time for school to start.

You can't imagine the thrill I had walking into the store

and heading for the racks of size 10. What a selection! I tried on everything that caught my eye. Each dress looked better than the one before. Every time I looked in the mirror, I murmured to myself, "You look great." I staggered happily out of the store, loaded down with bags and boxes of new blouses, skirts, dresses, and accessories.

For the debut of the new me, I attended church on the Sunday before the new school year began. I fixed up my hair and put on a yellow Irish linen dress, white high heels, and a long white lace mantilla. I didn't need much makeup because I was glowing with happiness and pride.

I waited until the church was almost full before I walked slowly to a front pew. I didn't pay much attention to the sermon because I was thinking about the rave comments I would receive outside. After Mass, in the churchyard, I basked in the compliments: "Is that really you?" "You look fantastic!" "What a beautiful slim woman you've become." I felt on top of the world. I didn't ever want to let that moment fade, and for days I replayed those compliments in my mind.

The night before my return to school, I was pumped up with excitement. I spread out different outfits on my bed, trying them on, taking them off, hoping to find the right look for the new me on the first day of school. I finally settled on a camel hair skirt, brown and white striped blouse, and a brown leather belt. A year earlier on the opening day of school, I had worn a black box-pleated skirt, dark blouse, and long black sweater. I had looked and felt drab. What a difference a year made.

Looking slim and trim, I strode into the school and made my presence known. I deliberately walked slowly by groups of students so they couldn't help but notice me. I heard whispers of amazement. Then the compliments began to fly. I enjoyed listening to every one of them, especially from Derek, the guy who had been afraid to take me out last year because he didn't want to be teased by his friends. He ran over to me and put his hands around my waist and said, "I can't believe it's you. You look great. I never knew you had such good-looking legs." All day in the halls, in the classroom, and in the cafeteria, classmates and teachers showered me with compliments.

In the days and weeks that followed, I felt things I had never known before—self-confidence, self-pride, and self-worth. The change in me was dramatic. The same girl who once spent her after-school hours sulking in her room now blossomed into a fun-loving, active teenager. The same girl who used to sit in the bleachers in P.E. class watching the girls play basketball now started as a guard. The same girl who sat home on the night of the junior prom the year before now had three invitations to the senior prom.

I had so much catching up to do, and it seemed as though there wasn't enough time in the day to do everything that I wanted. Each day seemed brighter than the last. I felt so good about myself because I had set a goal and reached it with hard work and determination. I never wanted to look back to the way I had been. The new me viewed the future with excitement and confidence. Everything I wanted was within my grasp, I thought.

Unfortunately, I quickly learned that being slim is no guarantee that life will hand you everything on a silver platter. You still must use your talents and skills and determination to succeed. Furthermore, I discovered that losing an extraordinary amount of weight doesn't mean you will stay slim forever.

After I graduated from high school, I realized that although I knew how to take the weight off, I didn't know how to keep it off because I didn't fully understand the principles of proper dieting and nutrition. As a result, I gained weight, lost it, and then put it right back on again. I became what most fat people are—a professional dieter. I knew what foods made me slim and what foods made me fat. I could look at any food on the table and tell you if it contained 23 calories or 230 calories. But I usually ignored the calories and pigged out.

By the time I was twenty-nine years old, I was married and the mother of four boys. And I was fat again. Very fat. I had gained 135 pounds since graduating from high school. I couldn't resist food. One morning, licking icing from my fingers, I told my husband over the phone that I had baked a double layer chocolate cake for dinner. As soon as I hung up, I ate a piece, and then another and another. By 3:00 P.M. I had eaten every crumb. Upset over what I had done, I hurried to the store, bought more mix, and baked another cake. It looked so good I ate two more slices before my husband came home. A few weeks later, I went to the doctor for a checkup. He told me, "If you don't lose weight, don't bother coming back." I thought, "I don't need to see this guy anymore. No one is going to tell me what to eat. I'll just find another doctor who will take my money." But a few months later when I took my chubby baby in for a checkup, the pediatrician said to me, "Do you want your son to be fat like you?" I didn't say anything, but inside I seethed with anger.

When I cooled down, I realized he was right. I took off my clothes and looked at myself in the mirror—all 275 pounds of blubber—and said to myself, "Oh, God, this is awful. You've got to diet."

But before I started, I walked into my favorite bakery, bought an apple cake, took it home, and wolfed it down. Then I ate every fattening food I could stuff into my face, knowing that the next day I would start another diet. Within the next eight months, I trimmed my weight in half, to 138 pounds.

When I went back to my doctor, he was delighted with my weight loss and saw how determined I was to stay slim. He suggested I start a class for overweight people because he thought I could be an inspiration to others. So I assembled a team of doctors, dietitians, and nutritionists who together created an easy-to-follow, nutritionally balanced diet plan to lose weight and keep it off. I founded a weight-loss program in Palm Beach County, Florida, and conducted diet classes for adults. The results they achieved were fantastic. Soon doctors throughout the area were advising their overweight patients to enter the program.

Although I helped show adults how to control their weight, my heart belonged to young people. I wanted to cry every time I saw an overweight young person because I knew he or she was going through the same misery I had experienced as a child. Finally, I decided to devote all my time and energy to helping overweight young people. I established Diet Encounter, a program of diet classes just for them—no adults allowed, not even parents.

Certainly one of the keys to the program's success has been the classes in which young people speak openly about their feelings, their problems, their goals. I have learned a lot from them. You can too. Throughout this book there are more than 150 personal remarks from these young people who share their experiences—sometimes good, sometimes bad. You will see that some names appear more than once. This is because kids were interviewed at different stages during their diets. What they have to say can help you as you embark on your own weight-loss challenge.

2
FAT ISN'T FUN

Being fat is a bummer.

Sometimes you want to cry or scream because you are so angry and frustrated. Sometimes you lock yourself in your room and never want to come out. Sometimes you feel so awful you just want to die.

You are not alone. Millions of overweight young people share similarly strong feelings—feelings, by the way, that almost always disappear when the fat disappears.

Like it or not, we live in a "thin-is-in" society that has no room for fat people. As a result, you are treated like a second-class citizen. Unfair? You bet it is. Nevertheless, it's a fact of life that isn't going to go away any time soon.

The only fat that most people think is cute is on babies. But when a child reaches school age, forget it. You probably found out the hard way what studies have already shown—students consider fat kids less likable than those who are thin or of average weight.

That sure doesn't help your self-confidence any, does it? Especially when you know deep down inside that you really are a likable person. Your feelings are hurt even further when you are taunted and teased by classmates, brothers, and sisters.

If someone says you are fat, what can you say? No comeback, no amount of fighting is going to change the fact that you are fat. All you have to do is look in the mirror and see the truth.

Growing up is tough enough without being saddled with the additional problem of being overweight. Let's assume you are like the young people who step into my diet classes for the first time.

You have been wounded so much by snide comments in school, at home, and in public that you avoid contact with others as much as possible. You don't even bother joining in all the activities that bring excitement and fun to young people. You stay cooped up in your house. You become afraid to try new things, afraid to speak your mind, afraid to develop your talents (unless they are talents that can be cultivated alone in your room, such as painting or writing poetry).

You begin to feel like a spectator in life rather than a participant. It's as if you are in the audience and everyone else is starring on stage. You feel like a social outcast. You suffer in silence, keeping it all bottled up inside.

Typically, you are ashamed of your body. If you are a boy, you cringe at the thought of taking off your shirt in public. In a touch football game of skins against the shirts, you would sit on the sidelines rather than take off your shirt to play for the skins. At the beach, you keep your shirt on no matter how hot it gets. You are embarrassed to take showers in gym class because your breasts look as big as your sister's.

If you are a girl, you shudder at the thought of exposing your upper arms or your thighs in public. You don't dare wear a two-piece bathing suit, halter top, or sleeveless dress. Bright colors are out because they draw attention to your body. You won't participate in any physically vigorous activity such as volleyball because your fat will jiggle.

So what does all this do to your self-esteem? It deflates

it like a pin-pricked balloon. You feel miserable and depressed. You feel as if you're not worth anything. You feel like a shadow—a big shadow standing nowhere. You become moody and no fun to be around. When you are asked to do something, you usually refuse. Your most-used sentence is "I can't," or "I won't," because either you are afraid to try or you don't have the energy.

It's easy to understand why you don't want to do anything. You are hampered by the burden of unneeded extra weight. Suppose you are 20 pounds overweight. That's like strapping onto your body five 1,500-page hardcover editions of *Webster's New Collegiate Dictionary* and wearing them twenty-four hours a day, seven days a week, without a second of relief. You end up so uncomfortable, so drained, that there is no way you can keep up physically with your friends. Because of that extra weight, you feel sluggish. You have no pep. You huff and puff whenever you climb stairs. Chances are good you suffer from stomachaches, backaches, and headaches.

Is this chapter sounding like a downer? It's supposed to read that way. Fat is not fun. It sure wasn't for me or the young people in my diet classes. I want you to read some of their comments, which are sometimes bitter and often sad. I've included their deep feelings and awful torment so you may realize that many fat young people think and act in much the same way as you do. Perhaps you can strongly identify with their problems. The comments in this chapter were made to me by young people before they began the diet.

One major point to remember is that nearly every one of these young people has since reached his or her weight goal. They are now winners. No matter how overweight they were or how much they suffered as fatties, they conquered their weight problems. Now they are enjoying their success as happy, confident young men and women who live life to the fullest.

Of course, it wasn't always that way. They felt hassled in school, at home, and in public. They also had trouble dealing with their own feelings and with developing friendships. Perhaps you have experienced similar dilemmas. Let's take a closer look at these common problem areas:

Problems at School

Life for a young fat person can seem pretty miserable in school. How many overweight students are chosen for the lead in the school play? How many overweight shortstops star on the baseball team? How many overweight girls are voted homecoming queen? Discrimination is not your only predicament. Stepping into the classroom can seem like walking through a mine field. You hope and pray you won't do something that will trigger an explosion of fat jokes.

Lydia, twelve, 38 pounds overweight: When I walk down the hall, the other kids shout "boom, boom" because I'm so fat. If I sneeze in class, the boys around me throw papers in the air and pretend a tornado went through. I hate going to class. I get so angry that I want to punch their lights out.

Bob, fifteen, 40 pounds overweight: I don't like getting up in front of the class because then everyone is looking at me. In social studies class, the teacher gave me a choice: either read my report in front of the class or take a lower grade. I took the lower grade.

Kevin, twelve, 34 pounds overweight: Once when we had to do five laps around the gym, I could do only one of them. The kids kept stepping on the backs of my tennis shoes and I kept falling down. Everyone laughed, even the coach. I started crying, so I had to stay after school for detention because the coach said I acted like a bad sport.

Barbara, eleven, 25 pounds overweight: I feel so bad all the time. The kids get in a circle around me and pinch me and punch me because I am fat. They know I won't tell the teacher. I keep quiet because I am afraid.

Diana, fifteen, 32 pounds overweight: I really looked forward to the school yearbook. When it came out, we all exchanged our books and wrote cute and funny things in them. I was fortunate because I had some good friends and they wrote nice things, which made me feel good. But then I noticed that under my picture someone had written "Weight Watchers failure." I threw the book away.

Problems at Home

How many times has your house been turned into a battleground? Your weight is the issue. In some households, parents argue with each other over their child's weight problem. In other homes, both parents gang up on the fat person, nagging and badgering him or her to go on a diet. Often a fight erupts when a brother or sister starts taunting and teasing. Conflict seems to swirl around the family of an overweight young person.

Michelle, thirteen, 44 pounds overweight: I don't remember any time that I wasn't fat. I was fat as a baby and I'm fat, fat, fat now. My sister says I'm an embarrassment to the whole family. I believe it, too. I get the worst household chores just because my sister doesn't want to ruin her long fingernails. Big deal. Who needs her?

Elyse, thirteen, 28 pounds overweight: My mother is always yelling at me to lose weight. Yet when we go shopping, she always picks out real stylish clothes that look great on a model but look terrible on me. She chose one green outfit that made me look like a stuffed pepper. I let her buy it just to satisfy her but I refused to wear it. Two weeks later as we were getting ready to attend a wedding, she insisted I wear the outfit but I refused. She got so mad she pulled it out of the closet and ripped it apart. I couldn't have cared less.

Problems in Public

There really is no way to dodge the slings and arrows of being fat. Once you step outside your house, you become fair game for all sorts of abuse. An insensitive comment from a stranger can hurt you, or you can suffer an embarrassing moment while shopping. It seems as though you can't go anywhere without getting zinged with a painful reminder that you are fat.

Thomas, thirteen, 44 pounds overweight: Let me tell you about the worst day of my life. I had to go shopping for school clothes with my mom. At the store I grabbed any pants I could find just to get it over with, because I hate shopping for clothes. In the dressing room I got the first pair on but I couldn't zip them up so I got down on the floor, lay on my back, and the zipper went up—but I couldn't get up. I must have looked like a turtle on my back. I started to sweat like crazy. Finally my mother came in and got me up, but then the zipper stuck and I couldn't get out of the pants. I was so nervous I almost fainted. I broke the zipper, peeled the pants off, hung them on a hook, and ran out of the store.

Melissa, thirteen, 41 pounds overweight: I wanted a new look so Mom took me to the hair salon. I wanted my hair cut short and feathered in the front. When I told the beautician how I wanted my hair done, she said, "Absolutely not. Your face is too fat. You're better off if it's parted down the middle." She said it so loud that everyone in the place could hear. Then she asked the others, "Isn't her face too fat for a short cut?" I wanted to die, I was so embarrassed. Mom stuck up for me but the beautician said that my face looked like a squirrel with chestnuts in its cheeks. I went home in tears.

Problems with Yourself

If you are like many fat young people, you suffer from a negative self-image because you view yourself the way you think others view you—as not being normal. Normal in this case means anyone who is not overly fat or terribly skinny. The teasing by your classmates, the discrimination in public, and your inability to keep up physically with the others because of your weight problem simply reinforce this negative view. Have you ever caught yourself thinking, "I'm no good" or "Who'd want anything to do with me?" or "I can't do anything right"? These thoughts are very common—and also very destructive. You can get caught in a whirlpool of depression, boredom, and frustration, which can suck you into one eating binge after another.

> *Joan, fourteen, 50 pounds overweight:* I am so fat, I know I am a real failure. I see pity in my mom's face. I hate myself. I want to be thin but I love food. I even sneak food into the bathroom, turn on the shower, and sit on the sink and eat and eat. I feel so guilty, so depressed.
>
> *Mark, fifteen, 45 pounds overweight:* I really hate myself and I am always in the pits. I feel cheated out of life and I also feel very, very guilty. Once I got so disgusted with myself that I

kept eating all day for three days straight. I really thought I was crazy. Then I felt guilty and angry with myself and I took it out on everyone else. I was very nasty.

Glenn, eleven, 22 pounds overweight: I am always mad at myself. I can tell people don't like me because everyone in school calls me names. I'm not normal. I hate myself so much I think everyone should hate me too. I won't tell my parents how I feel. I'm afraid they will agree with everyone else.

Margie, thirteen, 30 pounds overweight: I act weird around skinny people because I don't like the way I look. I'm different and I know it and that's why I don't like myself very much. I daydream that I'm thin and beautiful and have lots of friends. But that's all it is, just a dream. I look in the mirror and ask, "Why me?" I cry a lot.

Problems with Relationships

Why does it seem so hard to have friends and dates? One reason has to do with the way you view yourself. If you don't like yourself, then how do you expect others to like you? Another reason is that after years of being rejected and insulted because you are fat, you probably tend to shy away from people. By high school age, though, you want to be popular and go out on dates. But you learn that fat is not pretty; fat is not handsome.

Cindy, fifteen, 32 pounds overweight: I don't want anything to do with guys. Besides, who would want to go out with someone like me? I did fall in love for a week a few months back. I was at a dance at school and one of the football players asked me to dance with him. He wasn't a very good dancer but I didn't care. It felt so nice to be with a boy. That night I dreamed about him. I had a real crush on him. About a week later I found out that the only reason he asked me to dance was to win a ten-dollar bet with his buddies. Guys. Who needs them?

Phil, thirteen, 35 pounds overweight: I hang around with a bunch of guys and we play touch football and check things out at the mall. But I know the guys don't think much of me because I'm fat. It seems like every day they come up to me and say "How's it goin', Phil?" and then . . . bam! . . . punch me right in the arm. When I go home at night I'm black and blue. I just take it. Then there's the teasing. They call me the "walking garbage can." It hurts but I want to be around them. They are the only friends I have.

Sonia, sixteen, 38 pounds overweight: I'm fat and not very pretty so naturally I don't date. I got so tired of hearing about the other girls going on dates that I made up my own pretend boyfriend and wrote about him in my diary. My pretend boyfriend took me to the beach and to the movies and was always sending me poems or flowers. A real romantic. Maybe if I read over my diary enough times I'll begin to believe this romance really happened.

Laura, eleven, 24 pounds overweight: It seems like everyone around me is thin and they don't want anything to do with me. I get so nervous when kids call me names. I want to hide but I have no place to go. No one understands me and no one wants to. I care so much for people, but no one cares about me. No one loves a fat person—not even my parents.

Perhaps you are one of the few lucky overweight young people who is active and popular and has his or her act together. Congratulations. You've beaten the odds . . . for the moment. But let's take a peek at what you are likely to encounter in the near future. Do you think your good grades are automatically going to get you into college? Studies have shown that when personal interviews are required for college admission, fatties tend to be rejected more often than those who are not overweight. Things are no better when you look for a job. If the personnel manager of a business has to make a choice between hiring an overweight person and one who is equally qualified but isn't fat, guess who lands the job? This type of discrimination will haunt you throughout your life.

But of far more importance is the future of your health. Medical studies show that anywhere from 50 to 80 percent of overweight young people become overweight adults. And when you are an overweight adult, you increase your chances of diabetes, high blood pressure, stroke, and heart attack. Any one of these conditions can shorten your lifespan.

You don't deserve a future of discrimination and health problems. You deserve a better life. And a big step toward reaching that goal is to get rid of your fat problem. But before you look for the answers to achieving a safe and effective weight loss, first you should know the reasons why you are fat.

3

WHY YOU ARE FAT

Why are you fat?

Take a few minutes and think about that question. I'm sure you can come up with a good excuse. Notice I said "excuse" rather than "reason." I've heard one lame excuse after another that always sidesteps the truth. Here are some of the more common excuses. Is one of them yours?

"It's not my fault. I have a glandular problem." The thyroid gland, located at the base of the neck, plays a critical role in your growth and in the functioning of your body. If this gland is out of whack, you can turn into a blimp. However, since only a fraction of overweight young people suffer from any sort of glandular problem, you probably are not one of them. If your doctor *has* determined that you have a glandular problem, follow his or her advice about dieting.

"I'm big-boned so I have to eat more than most people." A person who has a large physique with broad shoulders would probably weigh more than someone who has a smaller skeletal frame, even if both are the same height.

The larger person may indeed have to eat more. But that's no excuse for being fat. You get fat from eating more calories than your body needs—no matter what your size.

"It's hard not to get fat because everywhere I look, I see fattening food." No doubt about it, high-calorie food tempts our taste buds dozens of times a day. Whole grocery-store aisles are devoted to sweetened, colored, gimmicky breakfast cereals. Junk food machines have invaded schools and public buildings. City thoroughfares are lined with belly-busting fast food joints. TV commercials assault us with commercials for fattening or sugary foods. But blaming Ronald McDonald, Colonel Sanders, and Tony the Tiger won't help you. No law says you must find your lunch in a junk food dispenser or dine at Hot Dog Heaven or snack on that yummy-looking dessert you saw advertised on TV. You can find wholesome, nutritious foods at the grocery store and in many restaurants. In fact, everything you need to stay healthy and slim was on this planet long before TV's first food commercial, the raising of the first golden arches, or the opening of the first supermarket.

"I can't help being fat. I inherited it from my parents." It sounds as if you have a strong case here, doesn't it? After all, according to *Public Health Bulletin*, there is a 40 percent chance that an overweight parent will raise an overweight child. The percentage doubles to 80 percent if both parents are fat. However, biological inheritance has little to do with it. Fatness is not inherited through genes the way blue eyes and dark hair are inherited. Nevertheless, there is a connection between overweight parents and their overweight children. Parents, grandparents, and other relatives can influence the way you eat, how much you eat, what you eat, and even your attitude toward eating. This is known as an eating pattern. You can grow up thinking that your family's eating pattern is normal, even if it isn't. For example, if no one in your family eats breakfast, then you would probably find it strange, after spending the night at a friend's house, to see your friend's family eating breakfast together. If your mother always provides big meat and potato dinners with homebaked bread, you would probably frown at the quiche and salad dinner at your friend's house. Fat parents often raise fat children because the children are merely reflecting the bad eating patterns of their parents. Aha! you say, that must prove your parents are to blame for your weight problem. Nope. I won't buy that argument. Unless your parents strapped you to a chair, pried open your mouth, and force-fed you fattening foods, you are the one who put that food in your mouth. You are old enough to know that taking an extra piece of Mom's cake or another helping of her casserole is going to tack on extra pounds.

"I'm fat because I have to eat what's put in front of me." Mom goes to a lot of trouble to prepare big meals so you eat lots of everything she cooks. Because you are starving by noon, you go ahead and eat the high-calorie food they serve in the school cafeteria. As a means of showing her love, Grandma bakes a platter of chocolate chip cookies and you please her by eating them all. At the restaurant, Dad warns, "Eat everything you order," and even though you are full, you clean your plate. Those are pretty tough situations for a young person to handle and it seems as though there is no choice but to eat. So it's everyone else's fault that you are overweight, right? Wrong. You get caught up in these situations because you haven't learned when to open your mouth at the right time—or when to shut it. Only after you understand the basic principles of a good diet do you learn when to shut your mouth to food. And only then do you learn how to open your mouth, to speak up without hurting feelings or creating arguments when food is placed in front of you. (I will discuss this matter in chapter 19, "Coping at Home.")

I reject the usual excuses for being overweight because

they don't focus on the one person who is ultimately responsible for the problem—*you*. Protest all you want, but the bottom line is that you make yourself fat. And here's how you do it:

- ✘ You eat too much.
- ✘ You eat the wrong food.
- ✘ You eat the wrong way.

Eating Too Much

Food provides energy for the body. This energy is measured in calories. If you consume more calories than your body burns, you gain weight. Girls should generally take in between 2,000 and 2,500 calories a day, while boys should have 2,500 to 3,000 calories per day. These figures are for normally active young people not on a diet. You use up most of these calories through physical activity such as dancing or bike riding and through growth and metabolism, the process that turns food into fuel to make your body work.

To maintain your ideal weight, you should consume the same number of calories that your body uses up. But this calorie number is different for each person. What is a proper amount of food for one person may be too much for you. Eating too much depends to a large extent on how many calories your body needs and how many it burns.

Let's assume you eat more than you should and consume 3,000 calories a day, and your body uses only 2,500 calories. That means 500 unused calories a day are stored up as fat. At the end of the week, the stored-up calories total 3,500—which happen to equal one pound of fat. In a year's time that could add up to 52 unneeded pounds.

Jerry, thirteen, 54 pounds overweight: I eat at least six meals a day. I have a big breakfast and then on my way to school I stop off at the store for a cupcake or candy bar. During lunch at school, I eat all the things that the other kids leave on their trays. Sometimes when I really like what's on the menu, I go through the cafeteria line with two trays and tell the lady that the second tray is for my friend. I go to a back table and eat both meals. After school, I eat another lunch, usually a sandwich, chips, and a soda. When Mom is cooking supper, I start nibbling at the food before she has a chance to put it on the table. She's a good cook, so I eat lots and lots, and then before bed I eat a snack of leftovers. Now ask me why I'm fat.

Debbie, fourteen, 47 pounds overweight: I love to eat. It's the great joy of my life, and I think about food all the time. My purse is full of candy bars, which I eat between classes. I try not to pig out at lunch at school because I don't want the other kids to call me a fat slob. But after school, I stop off at the bakery for a treat. At home I'm in the kitchen experimenting with new recipes. My family doesn't mind because they like the things I cook. I love big dinners. I love to make them and I love to eat them.

Jerry and Debbie are aware that they overeat, but many overweight young people have no concept of how much food they funnel down to their stomachs. Take Chuck's case, for example. He was an active fourteen-year-old who couldn't understand how he became 40 pounds overweight. "I eat a decent breakfast, the school lunch, dinner, and a few snacks, but I'm no monster eater. So why am I fat?" he asked. I told him to keep a daily record of everything he ate for one week to see if he was correct in claiming that he did not overeat. At the end of the week, we looked over his record and then I wrote down the calories of everything he ate. Here was a typical day for Chuck:

BREAKFAST

	CALORIES
2 slices fried bacon	86
2 fried eggs	198
1 slice of toast with 1 tablespoon jelly and 1 teaspoon butter	149
1 cup fresh orange juice	112

MID-MORNING SNACK

one 2-ounce candy bar with nuts	270

SCHOOL LUNCH

3 ounces turkey	150
½ cup mashed potatoes	98
1 roll with butter	109
½ cup green beans	22
1 cup whole milk	159
1 cupcake with icing	172

AFTER-SCHOOL SNACK

½ peanut butter and jelly sandwich	224
1 cup whole milk	159

DINNER

2 cups spaghetti and meatballs, with 2 teaspoons Parmesan cheese	665
2 pieces garlic bread	274
1 tossed salad with 2 tablespoons Italian salad dressing	226
one 8-ounce glass lemonade	107
1 cup ice cream	329

EVENING SNACK

20 potato chips	228
one 12-ounce bottle of cola	144
TOTAL	**3,881**

It may not appear that Chuck is a "monster eater." What he ate seems like a normal healthy appetite for any teenager, doesn't it? Nevertheless, he did consume more than 3,800 calories—about 1,000 more than he needed—and over 1,000 of those calories came from snacks. It's awfully easy to be fooled about how much we eat because we have a tendency to forget about all the snacks and drinks we consume. We also tend to forget how many calories are loaded in these foods and beverages.

Walking through your house could be an interesting eating experience. As you stroll through the living room, you grab a handful of peanuts in a bowl by the couch. In the dining room, you pop a caramel from a dish on a table. In the kitchen, you sneak a spoonful of ice cream from the freezer. On the desk in your bedroom is a bag of corn chips waiting to be opened.

See how easy it is to add extra pounds without even being fully aware of what you are doing? Let's assume you are maintaining your current weight. But if you eat a one-ounce chocolate candy bar (about 150 calories) every day, you could put on an additional 15 pounds by the end of the year. Eating only ten potato chips daily could add 11 pounds yearly. The same goes for munching on one oatmeal cookie every day.

How many times has this happened to you: You sit in front of the TV set with a big bag of potato chips in your lap and you start eating. About halfway through the show, your hand hits the bottom of the bag and you are startled to discover that you have eaten every single chip. You weren't conscious of how much you were eating.

You can even eat too much of a good thing. Margie was a thirteen-year-old who was about 30 pounds overweight, a problem she found difficult to understand because, she claimed, she ate only healthy, nutritious food and seldom touched junk food. As I did for Chuck, I asked Margie to keep a daily log of what and how much she ate for a week. The following week we studied the log.

True to her word, she didn't eat junk food and did eat plenty of fresh fruits and vegetables and all-natural products. However, the quantities she ate were enormous. Breakfast consisted of at least two bowls of cereal and three or four slices of whole wheat toast. Lunch included two tuna fish sandwiches and dinner centered around potatoes and chicken or rice and fish. But she always had at least two helpings, and her snacks throughout the day consisted of packages of peanuts or almonds and as many as four granola bars. When we tallied up the calories, they topped the 3,000 mark. She was overeating. The so-called right kinds of food don't guarantee you a slim, healthy life if you overeat. Remember, a calorie is a calorie no matter where it comes from.

Eating the Wrong Food

The typical American teenager has one of the worst diets in the world. In many ways, some poor children in Latin America eat better: tortillas, beans, cheese, chicken, an occasional egg, and fresh fruits and vegetables, which together provide vital protein, carbohydrates, minerals, and vitamins. Now compare that to the young American who wolfs down sugar-coated breakfast cereal, nutritionless soda, additive-loaded canned spaghetti, greasy cheeseburgers, salted pretzels, and chemical-laden frozen dinners. Yuck!

> *Peter, fourteen, 46 pounds overweight:* To me, fruits and vegetables and salads are nothing more than health foods. I don't like them and I won't eat them. When I see skinny people eating yogurt, I feel sorry for them because they don't know what they are missing. Food is to be enjoyed and I enjoy burgers and fries and soda at lunch. I like cupcakes

and cookies so I eat them. And at night I always have chips or pretzels and a soda.

Dale, twelve, 16 pounds overweight: My parents tell me I have a sweet tooth. I can't help it. I just have to have something sweet in my mouth—candy, gum, cookies. It doesn't matter. I have a candy bar stash in my closet because my parents are trying to crack down on the sweets at home. I can't ever picture giving up candy.

The food you eat affects your health, your appearance, your energy, your growth, and of course, your weight. Eating too much of the wrong foods—and not enough of the right ones—can make you feel sluggish and can make you fat.

The best way to avoid trouble like this is to consume the proper amount of nutrients. These are chemical substances obtained from food during digestion. Food is made up of different nutrients needed for growth and energy. Each nutrient has one or more specific jobs to perform in the body and usually does its best work when teamed with other nutrients. To maintain good health, you need about fifty nutrients a day because they help build and maintain your body cells, regulate your body processes, and supply energy. Since no single food supplies all fifty nutrients, you should eat a variety of foods daily, especially those that contain these ten major nutrients:

Protein. Except for water, you have more protein than any other substance in your body. It's found in the cells of muscles, blood, and bone and is vital to the growth of new tissue and the repair of existing tissue. Important sources of protein are meat, poultry, fish, cheese, milk, dried beans, peas, lentils, and nuts.

Carbohydrates. The starches, sugars, and fiber in foods from plants are carbohydrates and provide you with energy. Among major sources of carbohydrates are fruits, grain products, and starchy vegetables like potatoes, lima beans, and corn.

Fat. It is part of the structure of every cell in your body. Stored body fat insulates you and is also a source of energy. You find fats in shortening, oil, butter, margarine, salad dressings, and many meats.

Vitamin A. It assists in the formation and maintenance of your skin, helps increase your resistance to infection, and promotes healthy eye tissue. Vitamin A, also known as retinol, can be found in orange fruits and vegetables, dark green leafy vegetables, and liver.

Vitamin C. It holds body cells together, strengthens blood vessels, helps heal wounds and broken bones, and increases resistance to infections. Also known as ascorbic acid, Vitamin C is obtained from citrus fruits, dark green leafy vegetables, and tomatoes.

Vitamin B_1 (Thiamin). It helps promote a proper appetite and a healthy central nervous system. Important sources of thiamin are lean pork, nuts, oatmeal, and fortified cereal products like Total and Special K.

Vitamin B_2 (Riboflavin). It helps with the production of energy within body cells and promotes healthy skin, eyes, and clear vision. Major sources of riboflavin are fortified grain products, such as some macaroni and bread, as well as milk, yogurt, and liver.

Niacin. This vitamin helps you digest your food, promotes healthy skin, and aids your nervous system. Significant sources of niacin are meat, poultry, fish, liver, and fortified cereal products.

Calcium. This mineral helps form and give strength and structure to your bones and teeth. About 99 percent of the calcium in your body is in your skeleton. Calcium also helps your blood to clot. It is obtained from milk and milk products, sardines, and collard, kale, mustard, and turnip greens.

Iron. It combines with protein to form hemoglobin, the red substance in your blood that carries oxygen to and carbon dioxide from the cells. Iron helps prevent fatigue and increases your resistance to infection. Major sources of iron are enriched farina, liver, and red meat.

Generally speaking, if you eat foods rich in these ten nutrients every day, you will automatically be consuming sufficient amounts of the other forty nutrients. That is why it is so important to eat a balanced diet. (A balanced diet does not mean holding a cupcake in each hand.)

On a balanced diet, you eat a variety of foods from these four major food groups:

Dairy. These foods supply calcium, protein, and vitamin B_2 and include milk and milk products, such as cheese, cottage cheese, yogurt, and ice cream and ice milk.

Protein-Rich Foods. Foods in this group include meat, poultry, fish, eggs, dried beans, and nuts. In addition to protein, they supply niacin, iron, and thiamin.

Fruits and vegetables. These foods supply vitamins A and C, and most are low in calories and are filling.

Grain and fiber. Foods in this group supply carbohydrates, thiamin, iron, and niacin. They also contain fiber, a substance that makes food chewy and acts like a sponge in your stomach, soaking up liquid so you feel full and don't eat so much. Sources of this food group are grains such as wheat, rice, and corn, cereals, whole wheat bread, grits, noodles, and pasta.

You can expect to be fat if your diet is not balanced and is overloaded with too many fattening foods. Ideally, of the food you eat, 15 to 20 percent of the calories should be in the form of proteins, 50 to 55 percent carbohydrates, and 30 percent fats.

Most young people consume more than 40 percent of their calories in the form of fat—from 800 to 1,200 calories of fat per day. That's too much. Every ounce of fat contains more than twice the calories of an ounce of protein or carbohydrates. So what happens when you eat lots of foods with fat? You end up fat.

The same thing can happen when you eat too much sugar. White refined sugar, the kind in your sugar bowl, is not really a food because it has no vitamins, no useful minerals, and no protein. The only benefit it offers is that it makes food taste sweet. When sugar and sweetened foods make up a large part of your intake of calories, they replace other foods that offer vitamins, minerals, and proteins. Furthermore, you can acquire such a craving for sweets that you end up eating more and more, which leads to consuming greater amounts of calories than you realize.

Soda pop, bagged and boxed snacks, candy, ice cream, pastries, and presweetened cereals are made up mainly of "empty" calories. By that I mean they are foods with little or no nutritional value—no vitamins, minerals, or protein to help nourish the body. For example, if you eat 200 calories of "tummy yummies," your body can't do much with the calories except store them as fat. However, if you eat the same amount of calories of fish, for instance, your body receives needed vitamins, minerals, and protein.

Don't believe all that hype about sugar being the best source of energy. If you are tired, a good dose of sugar from a couple of candy bars may perk you up temporarily, but you'll soon feel more listless—and even hungrier. This is because of chemical reactions that sugar causes in your body.

Soft drinks are loaded with sugar. Do you know what's in a twelve-ounce bottle of cola? Flavored water and seven teaspoons of sugar. In a year's time, the average American teenager consumes nearly five hundred bottles of soft drinks, two hundred pieces of chewing gum, and over twenty pounds of candy.

Another nasty source of sugar is presweetened breakfast cereal. Take your box of presweetened cereal down from the shelf and look at the label. What's the first ingredient you usually see? Sugar. The law requires that the ingredients be listed in order of quantity with the largest single ingredient first. What the label tells you is that your cereal contains more sugar than any other ingredient.

People with a weight problem often eat too much sodium. The main source of sodium is table salt. Too much sodium in your diet could cause high blood pressure. Sodium also helps retain unnecessary amounts of water in your body. But even if you don't use much table salt, you still may be eating too much sodium because it is found in so many packaged and precooked foods such as smoked meat, luncheon meats (like bologna), corned beef, hot dogs, sausage, pickles, olives, condiments (like ketchup and mustard), potato chips, and pretzels.

You don't develop a weight problem by eating the wrong kinds of food for a few days. You become overweight from eating fatty, nutrition-poor foods over a long period of time.

Eating the Wrong Way

It's pretty hard to become fat without having developed the wrong attitude toward food and without having learned a bunch of bad eating habits.

Let's tackle attitude first. To many fat young people, food is their best friend, their security blanket, their reason to enjoy life. Ever since you were a toddler you learned that a sweet treat can stop your tears. Remember when you scraped your knee and Mommy gave you a cookie to make it feel all better? So now you use food to comfort yourself when you are depressed or angry. You've learned that food can be a reward: After winning a debate in speech class, you decide to reward yourself with a hot fudge sundae on your way home from school.

If you are really fat, it's partly because you have fallen head over heels in love—with food, that is. You can't go anywhere or do anything without eating or at least thinking about food. Your life, like mine as a child, revolves around food. (I was a chocaholic. I had to have my chocolate fix or I was miserable. I used to have dreams about being locked overnight in the Hershey candy bar factory, swimming in a vat of pure chocolate. The only kisses I wanted were the ones wrapped in foil.) Maybe to you, Fantasy Island means owning your own private Dunkin' Donuts. Heaven is a white marble Burger King serving only one customer forever—you. The perfect world would abound in ice cream mountains, cola lakes, French fry forests, and pastry canyons.

Don, seventeen, 87 pounds overweight: I always viewed food as my best friend. But recently I realized it wasn't a friend at all. Food doesn't talk to you. It doesn't listen to your problems. It doesn't laugh or cry or give you advice. It gains your trust by comforting you at first but it ends up giving you all sorts of problems. It doesn't solve the problems. It only makes you more miserable the more you are around it.

Carmen, fifteen, 62 pounds overweight: I know why I'm fat. I eat for the sake of eating. It's just a habit with me. No matter where I go or what I do, I am always eating. Really, I don't eat big, fancy meals at all. I just eat throughout the day. Between classes, on the school bus, talking on the phone, playing records. It seems I can't even carry on a conversation unless I have food near me. I guess it's like Linus's security blanket in the Peanuts comic strip.

Can you see how Carmen's attitude toward food has played a major part in making her fat? Don't make food more than it is. If you can derive pleasure from eating, wonderful. But understand that its main purpose is to provide fuel for your body. You shouldn't live to eat. You should eat to live.

Often the wrong attitudes toward food lead to the development of bad eating habits. These are learned habits that you follow every time you eat—and they are bad because they contribute to your weight problem. How many bad eating habits do you have? Answer the following twenty-five questions with a simple yes or no.

EATING HABITS QUIZ

1. Do you automatically eat a snack of something other than a piece of raw fruit or vegetable when you come home from school?
2. Do you raid the refrigerator whenever you feel angry, depressed, bored, or nervous?
3. Do you eat while talking on the phone, doing homework, or watching TV?
4. When you help prepare dinner, do you sample the food before it is served?
5. Do you eat in rooms other than the kitchen or dining room?
6. Are you a member of the "clean plate club"?
7. Do you finish eating in less than twenty minutes?

8. Do you automatically put salt on your food before tasting it?
9. Do you usually eat second helpings?
10. Do you usually eat bread and butter with dinner?
11. Do you eat a dessert after almost every dinner?
12. Do you usually accept food when it's offered at a friend's house?
13. When you accomplish something such as getting an A on a test, do you reward yourself with a sweet treat?
14. Do you snack on junk food throughout the day?
15. When you are enjoying an activity such as skating, going to the movies, or playing at the video game arcade, are you eating at the same time?
16. Do you eat candy or peanuts or other snacks because they are kept within easy reach in the house?
17. When people tease you about your weight, or when you are nagged by your parents, do you tend to eat more?
18. When you are happy or excited, do you find yourself snacking?
19. Do you drink sodas with your meals?
20. Do you skip breakfast?
21. Do you automatically sprinkle sugar on your cereal?
22. If you see someone else snacking, do you then find something to eat too?
23. When you are at a fast food restaurant, do you usually order the biggest portions, such as a jumbo drink, double order of fries, or a triple burger?
24. Do you nibble on goodies while grocery shopping?
25. Do you finish off the leftovers on the dinner table instead of putting them away for another meal?

How did you score on this quiz? For every yes answer give yourself a slap on the wrist because each yes answer points to a bad eating habit. The more of these bad eating habits you have, the more likely you are to suffer from a weight problem.

You weren't born with these habits. You learned them until they became so routine in your everyday life that you weren't even aware of them. (In chapter 10, "The Good Eating Habit," I will show you how to unlearn these bad eating habits.)

There are two bad eating habits that deserve special attention. The first is skipping breakfast. Are you one of those people who think that you can cut down on calories by not eating breakfast? Well, my friend, let me set you straight. You end up *gaining* weight. Here's why:

When you avoid breakfast, you become famished by lunchtime, so you overeat. You consume more calories at one sitting than you would have with a simple breakfast and a regular lunch. You cram all the day's eating—lunch, snacks, dinner, and a bedtime treat—into an eight-to-ten-hour period rather than spreading it throughout a thirteen-to-fifteen-hour period. When food is consumed only in the last half of the day, the calories cannot be metabolized very efficiently because so much food is entering the body in a short period of time. As a result, the calories are stored as fat. So start eating a decent breakfast every day.

Another major bad eating habit is eating too fast. By gobbling food down at pie-eating-contest speed, you don't give your stomach time to yell, "Enough!" Only when you are finally bursting at the seams do you suddenly realize that you should have quit after the first helping. But by then it's too late. You have exceeded the feed limit.

Jake, fifteen, 38 pounds overweight: I'm fat because it's easy to eat your problems away. I can eat a large pizza by myself. When the family goes to the pizza place, I eat those slices real fast so I can be sure of getting the most pieces.

Slowing down allows you the luxury of knowing when to stop—if you listen to your body. To be in tune with your body, you must understand the difference between appetite and hunger. When you are hungry, your empty stomach sends a message to the brain saying, "Hey, send some food down here. I don't care what kind of food it is just as long as it fills me up." Because your stomach doesn't have taste buds, it will be satisfied with most any kind of food. An appetite develops when you think about food and crave a certain taste—such as French fries, ice cream, or candy—whether or not you are hungry. It's all in your mind, not in your belly.

Let's say Terri bolts down a double cheeseburger at her favorite fast food joint. It's so delicious she orders another one. But halfway through her second cheeseburger, Terri realizes she doesn't really want it. She ate more than she should because she didn't listen to her stomach. Instead she let her appetite control her actions. Here's what happened: Terri ate her first sandwich so fast that her stomach didn't have enough time to signal the brain that the stomach was full and satisfied. And because of her appetite—the desire for the taste of a cheeseburger—she ordered a second one. Only after she was halfway through eating cheeseburger number two did her brain receive the stomach's message that it was full. Had Terri eaten slowly, she never would have ordered the second cheeseburger.

Slow down when you eat. And before reaching for a second helping ask yourself, "Am I still hungry?" Get in tune with your stomach for the answer.

Now that you've admitted that you became fat by eating too much, eating the wrong foods, and eating the wrong way, what are you going to do about it?

Going on the Diet

4
MAKING UP YOUR MIND

There comes a time when you get so angry, so depressed, so frustrated, and so teased about being fat that you are ready to change your life. You are ready to lose weight.

Katey, fourteen, 32 pounds overweight: I woke up one morning very depressed and looked in the mirror. I thought it was going to crack. I was ugly—fat cheeks, fat arms, greasy hair, pimply face. God, I was a mess. I looked in that mirror for fifteen minutes and couldn't find one thing I liked. Then I let my eyes go out of focus and I had a mental picture of a thin, very pretty girl. It was the person I wanted to be. Right then and there I made up my mind to lose weight.

Craig, twelve, 21 pounds overweight: I ate food like crazy. I was a mean eating machine. One night I was putting away a whole large double cheese and pepperoni pizza when I began to choke on a real big piece. I couldn't breathe. I thought my eyes were going to pop out of my head. Finally the piece went down but my throat was sore for a day. It really scared me and taught me a lesson about the way I eat. I decided to go on a diet right away.

Marsha, sixteen, 42 pounds overweight: I hit an all-time low at a slumber party. The only reason I was invited was because it was my cousin who was throwing the party. Well, everyone was talking about boys and falling in love and I felt so left out because when you are fat like me you don't have boyfriends. So I stayed in the kitchen and fixed food for everyone. I ate and ate until I had to call my father to come and get me because I got sick. I knew I had to change because I couldn't go on living this way. Within a couple of days I began to diet.

Cindy, fifteen, 32 pounds overweight: I was at school, and when I went to bend over to pick up a pencil from the floor, I split my slacks right in the seat. I was so embarrassed. I had a friend walk directly behind me to the office and I called my mother and asked her to bring me another pair of slacks. I knew then I had better go on a diet because I was wearing my mother's slacks—and she's real fat.

Sissy, ten, 27 pounds overweight: We were playing dodge ball and all the kids wanted me in the middle so they could have an easy target. They said no one could miss hitting me because I was so big. I couldn't help it, I cried. I hate being teased. That's why I went on a diet.

You don't have to be hounded forever by the problems you have suffered as a fat person. You can change your life. Granted, it won't be easy and it will take time, but you can do it.

I wish I could give this book to every fat young person and say, "Read this, and by the time you finish it, you will be thin." Unfortunately, nobody can make you thin. The doctor can't. Your parents can't, and neither can your friends. Only you can make yourself lose weight. You must shoulder the responsibility of this diet because it is your body. And nobody knows your body better than you do. You must care about yourself, your body, your feelings. You must care about losing weight.

Don, seventeen, 87 pounds overweight: Just because you are fat, that doesn't make you less of a person. You are a person for who you are inside, not how you look in jeans. You must try to like yourself and accept yourself as a person if you are ever to do anything about your weight problem.

Losing weight takes hard work. It's much like school. Unless you're a teenage Einstein, you have to work very hard researching and writing a social studies term paper in order to earn an A. In dieting, you must make a similarly strong effort. You also must show desire, determination, and confidence.

So what if you failed on other diets? That was in the past. Perhaps you dieted because your parents nagged you to death. Or the doctor ordered you to do it. It wasn't your decision. Maybe you tried a diet that was geared for an adult, or you followed some unworkable fad diet. Those other diets were just bad experiences. Put them out of your mind and stop feeling guilty that you failed on them. Try something that is guaranteed to work. Try something for yourself.

Daniel, thirteen, 40 pounds overweight: Mom made me go on a diet and I hated it. I lost 18 pounds but I couldn't hack it anymore so I quit and then I gained 30 pounds. You can't diet until you are ready to diet. You have to want to do it for yourself.

Like many young people who first come to my diet classes, Laura did not do so voluntarily. The first time I talked to Laura, she told me she didn't want to be seen with all the other fat people in my class. "I'm here because my mother made me come," she told me. "I don't think this diet will work anyway."

"Do you want to be slim? Do you want to wear beautiful clothes?" I asked.

"Yes, more than anything."

"Are you willing to try a diet that I promise will work?"

"I guess so. I'll give you a couple of weeks."

"Don't give *me* anything. Give *yourself* all the time it takes to make this diet work."

She did. In four weeks, Laura lost 13 pounds. A month later she took off another 8 pounds and reached her target weight.

Let's say you've read this far and are thinking of telling your parents, "Okay, I read the first few chapters. How much more do I have to read?" If that's the case, then put this book on the shelf. Don't read any further because you're not ready to make the commitment to lose weight. I say this because I'm not going to convince you to lose weight. If I have to persuade you, I can almost guarantee that you won't make it through the diet. You must have the desire and make the effort or it won't work. All I can do is show you how you can lose weight. The rest is up to you.

You say you have the desire? You want to make the commitment? You're tired of being fat? Okay, then go ahead and finish the book. Follow the guidelines and you'll see the results. You'll be so amazed that you will have more determination to succeed than ever before. So tell yourself, "Do it now!" You know as well as I that the longer you wait, the harder it's going to be for you, because a few months down the road, you will have put on another 10 or 15 pounds.

Don't start this diet unless you're fired up and ready to take on the world with a positive attitude. If you are thinking, "Another day, another diet," you're not ready. I want you to believe that each day on this diet will be a step closer to a new and better you. This diet is not a punishment. It's a plan for a happier, healthier life. You must diet for the most important person in your life—you. You have nothing to lose but your weight. And you have lots to gain (except pounds). You deserve to feel good about yourself and your body.

Heidi, thirteen, 35 pounds overweight: Dieting was my first real challenge. I started to diet with a friend of mine and I was out to lose more than she could. But then something happened to me. I didn't care about my friend's weight. I wanted to prove to myself that I could actually accomplish something that was very difficult. Each week brings me more success and that makes me feel very happy.

Mardee, fourteen, 26 pounds overweight: When a slender girl walks by in a tight-fitting pair of Calvin Klein's, I don't go around saying, "Gee, I wish that was me." Instead I say, "That will be me soon." I can look just as wonderful in those jeans as she can.

Don't just wish yourself thin. Visualize it. Believe it. Picture yourself strolling in a sleek new swimsuit . . . or dancing the night away with a dreamy date . . . or crossing the finish line in a ten-kilometer race.

To help free your imagination, try this simple exercise: First, find a quiet place to relax, such as your bedroom or under a tree in your backyard. Sit in a comfortable position and close your eyes. Now tense up all your muscles, count to three, and then relax. Do this five times. Next, inhale slowly and deeply through your nose and exhale through your mouth. Do this five times. Now picture a long hallway leading to double doors. As you approach, the doors swing open. There on the other side is a nice-looking, well-groomed, slender person—the person you intend to look like when you reach your weight goal. Study the person. The hair. The eyes. The smile. The tailored fit of the clothes. The confident tone of voice. This is the person you will become.

To help you create that image in your mind, look for

inspiration. You might find it in a photo of your favorite movie star or baseball player, or your best friend, or your brother or sister. But be realistic and don't try to copy somebody. After all, you are a unique person—there is no one else in the whole world exactly like you—so try to picture in your mind how you will look when you reach your goal.

That image can be turned into reality if you are willing to work hard and stick to the diet. Let me level with you though: I can't promise that once you reach your weight goal you will be the next class president or the star quarterback or win the title role in the school play. But I can promise you that the opportunities to do these things—or whatever else your goals are—will be much greater. They will be within your grasp not only because you will have become thin but also because you will have proven to yourself that you can succeed. You will discover that if you want something badly enough and work hard enough, you can do almost anything. Losing weight—and keeping it off—will be one of the most difficult things you will ever accomplish. In comparison, other goals may seem much easier to reach.

If you are willing to make a commitment to lose weight, then I am ready to make a pact with you. It's the same one I make with each person who begins one of my classes. It goes like this: "I promise to help you reach your weight goal if you promise to try very hard to follow the You Can Do It! Kids Diet." So is it a deal?

5

GET READY, GET SET...

You probably are very anxious to start the diet. Be patient. You can't just make up your mind one day and then start the diet the very next day. Dieting is serious business and it requires some planning and preparation to help you achieve success. So before you start the diet, do the following:

Visit your doctor. With a complete physical examination, your physician can rule out the slight chance that your weight problem is caused by a glandular condition. The doctor can also determine if you should take a vitamin or mineral supplement, especially if you've been eating nutritionally poor food up to now. Although the diet supplies you with the necessary daily requirements of vitamins and minerals, it's wise to take a daily over-the-counter multiple vitamin during the first month as your body adjusts to a healthy eating plan. Show your doctor the basics of this diet on pages 67–95 and discuss it with him or her. *Remember, do not go on this diet without your doctor's consent.*

Set a weight goal. Be realistic. Don't set your goal too high. With your doctor, study the growth charts on pages 57–60. They can give you a general idea of how much you should weigh. To figure out approximately what you should weigh, first find the percentile (one of the curved lines on the growth charts) closest to your height on the height-for-age chart. To do this, find your age on the scale at the bottom of the chart and draw a line up to the top of the chart. (The age scale is marked off in half years, so round off your age to the nearest half year. In other words, if you are 13 years, 4 months old, round it off to 13½.) Then find your height on the scale at the left of the chart and draw a line across the chart. Where the two lines intersect, mark an **x** with a pencil. The curved line closest to your mark is the percentile. Next, turn to the weight-for-age chart. Again, find your age at the bottom of the chart and draw a line up to the top of the chart. Where the line intersects the same percentile as that of your height, mark an **x** with a pencil. Next, draw a horizontal line from the mark to the weight scale at the left of the chart. The point where the line intersects the weight scale tells you in a general sense what you should weigh. But that is not necessarily your weight goal. In fact, you may not need to lose as much weight as you think—if you are still growing. Losing a substantial amount of weight may take several months, so you must make an adjustment in your weight goal to allow for any anticipated growth spurts.

To illustrate, let's say twelve-year-old Amy is 4 feet 10 inches (58 inches) tall and weighs 120 pounds. According to the charts, her height is in the twenty-fifth percentile, but her weight is in the ninetieth percentile. To figure out approximately what her weight goal should be, she must find the twenty-fifth percentile in weight for girls her age. According to the chart, her weight should be about 80 pounds. However, we must take into consideration that Amy still has some growing to do. As a result, she doesn't

GIRLS FROM 2 TO 18 YEARS OLD

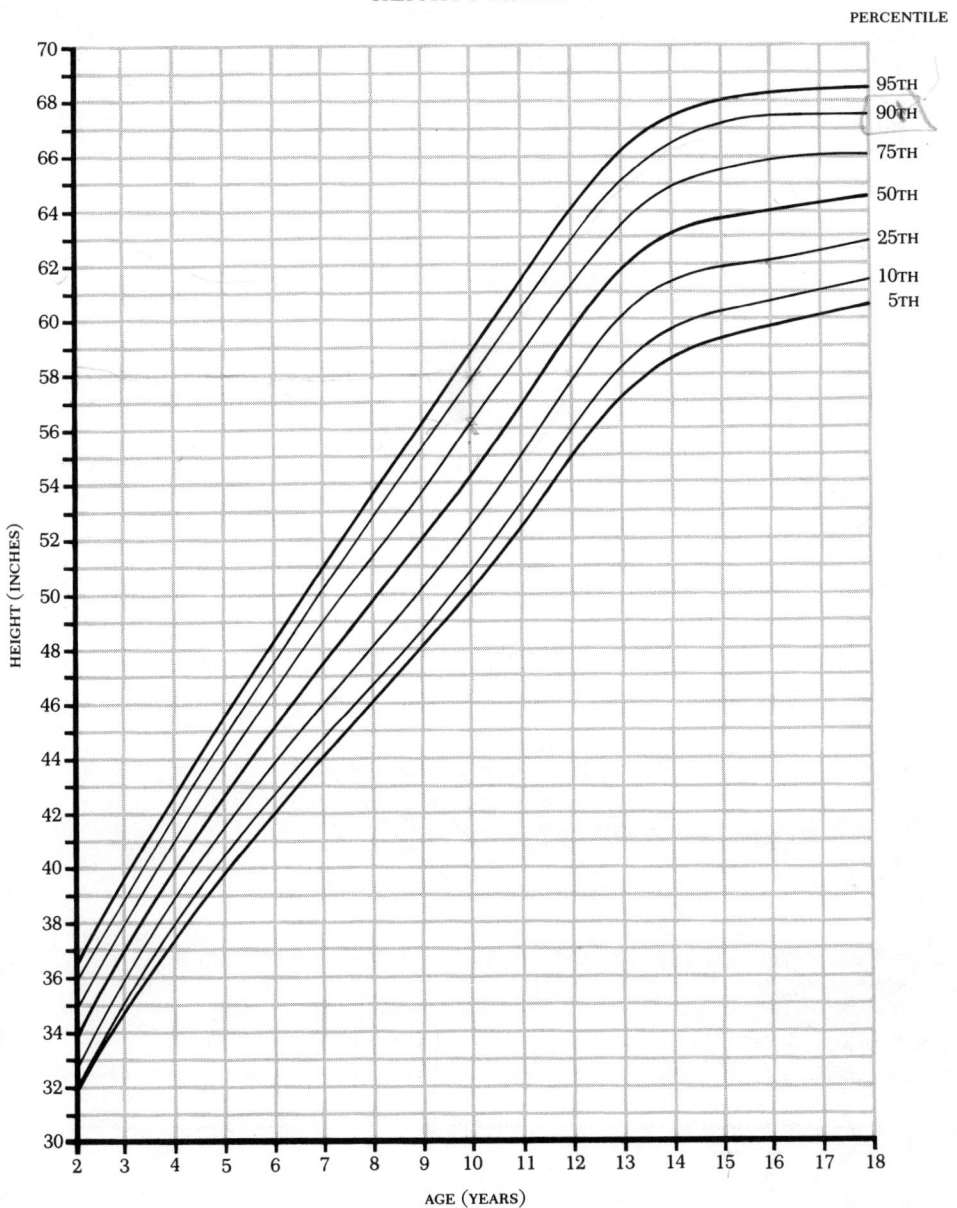

HEIGHT FOR AGE

PERCENTILE
- 95TH
- 90TH
- 75TH
- 50TH
- 25TH
- 10TH
- 5TH

HEIGHT (INCHES)

AGE (YEARS)

Credit: Department of Health and Human Services

GOING ON THE DIET

GIRLS FROM 2 TO 18 YEARS OLD

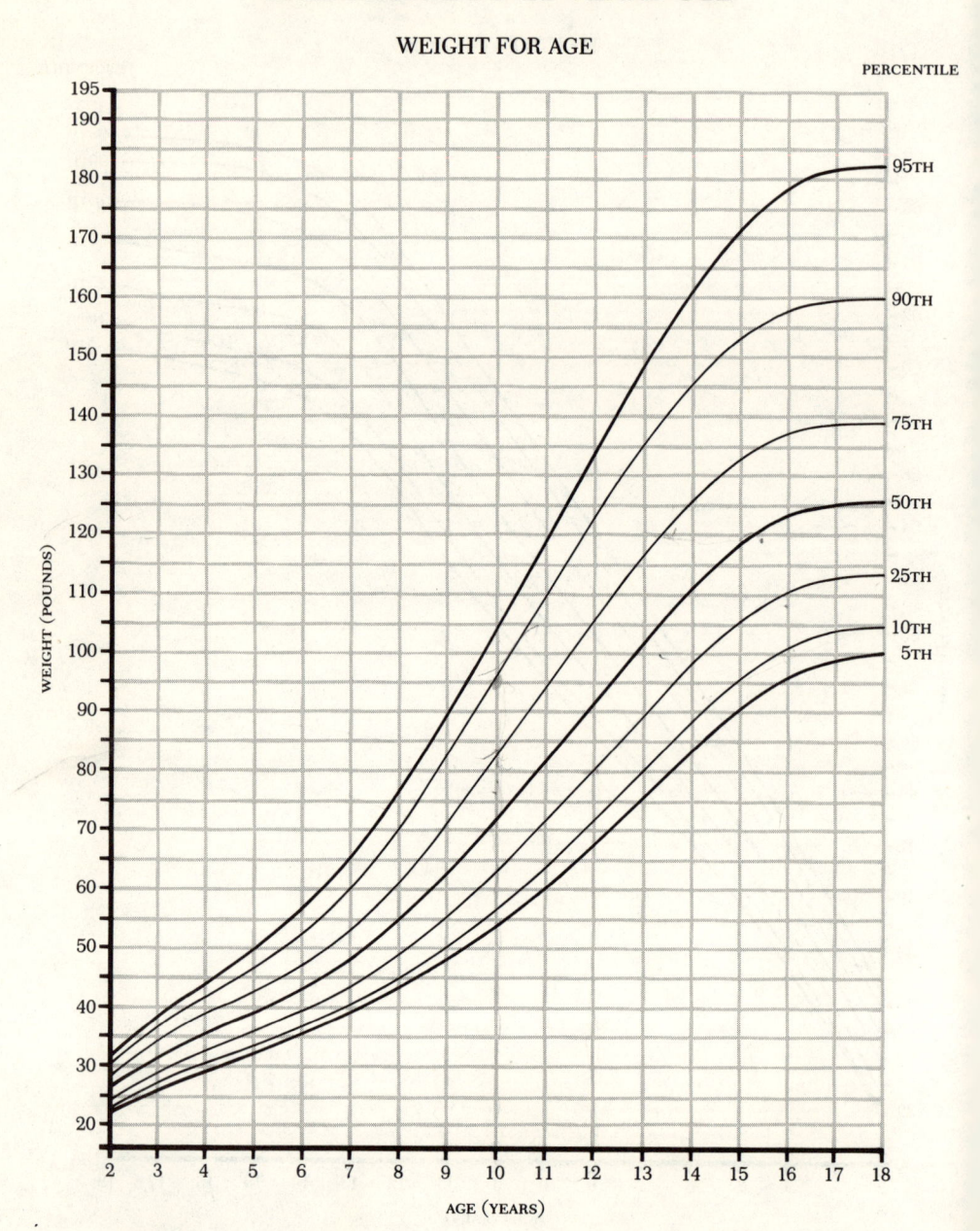

WEIGHT FOR AGE

PERCENTILE

WEIGHT (POUNDS)

AGE (YEARS)

- 95TH
- 90TH
- 75TH
- 50TH
- 25TH
- 10TH
- 5TH

Credit: Department of Health and Human Services

GET READY, GET SET . . . **59**

BOYS FROM 2 TO 18 YEARS OLD

HEIGHT FOR AGE

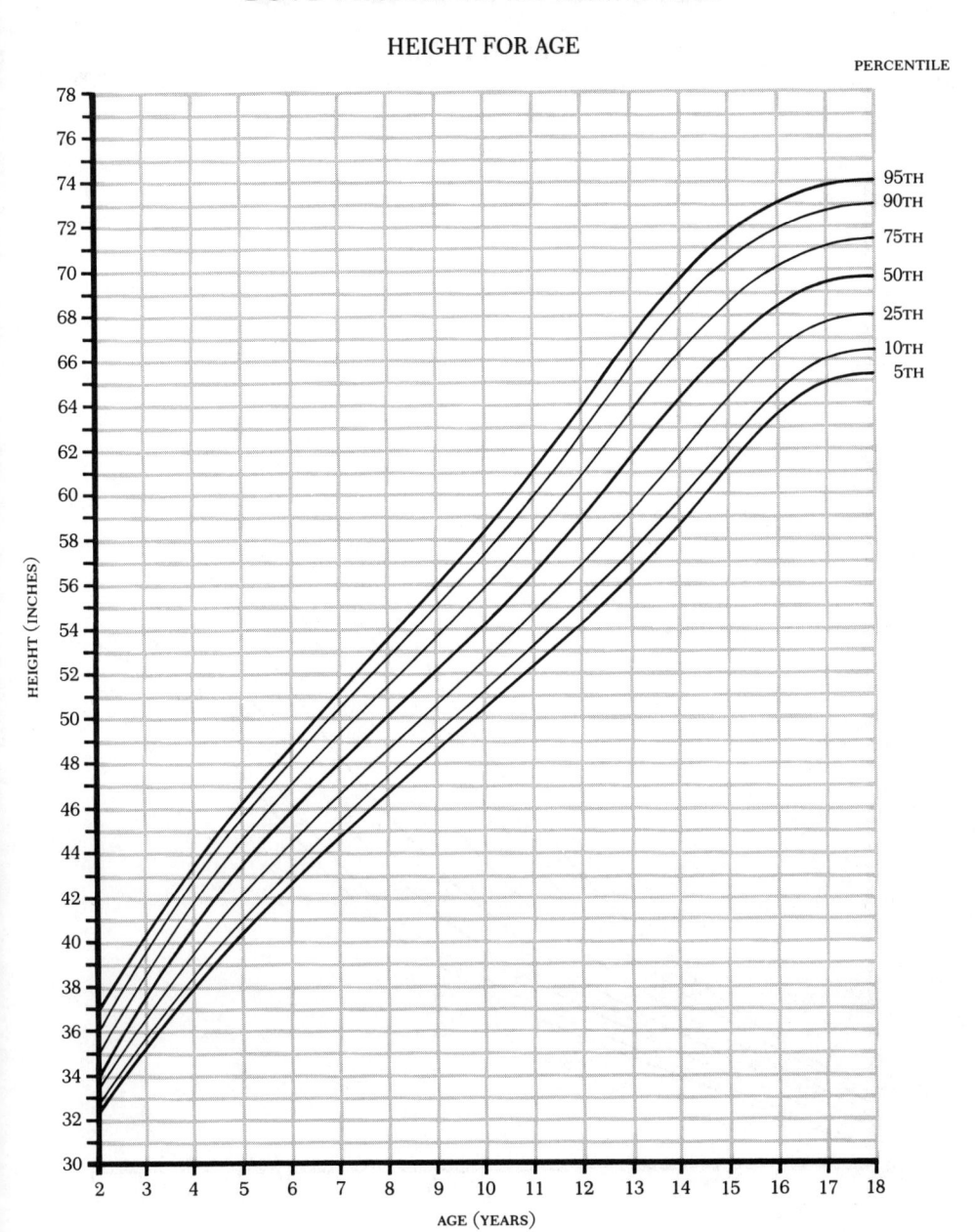

PERCENTILE: 95TH, 90TH, 75TH, 50TH, 25TH, 10TH, 5TH

HEIGHT (INCHES) vs AGE (YEARS)

Credit: Department of Health and Human Services

60 GOING ON THE DIET

BOYS FROM 2 TO 18 YEARS OLD

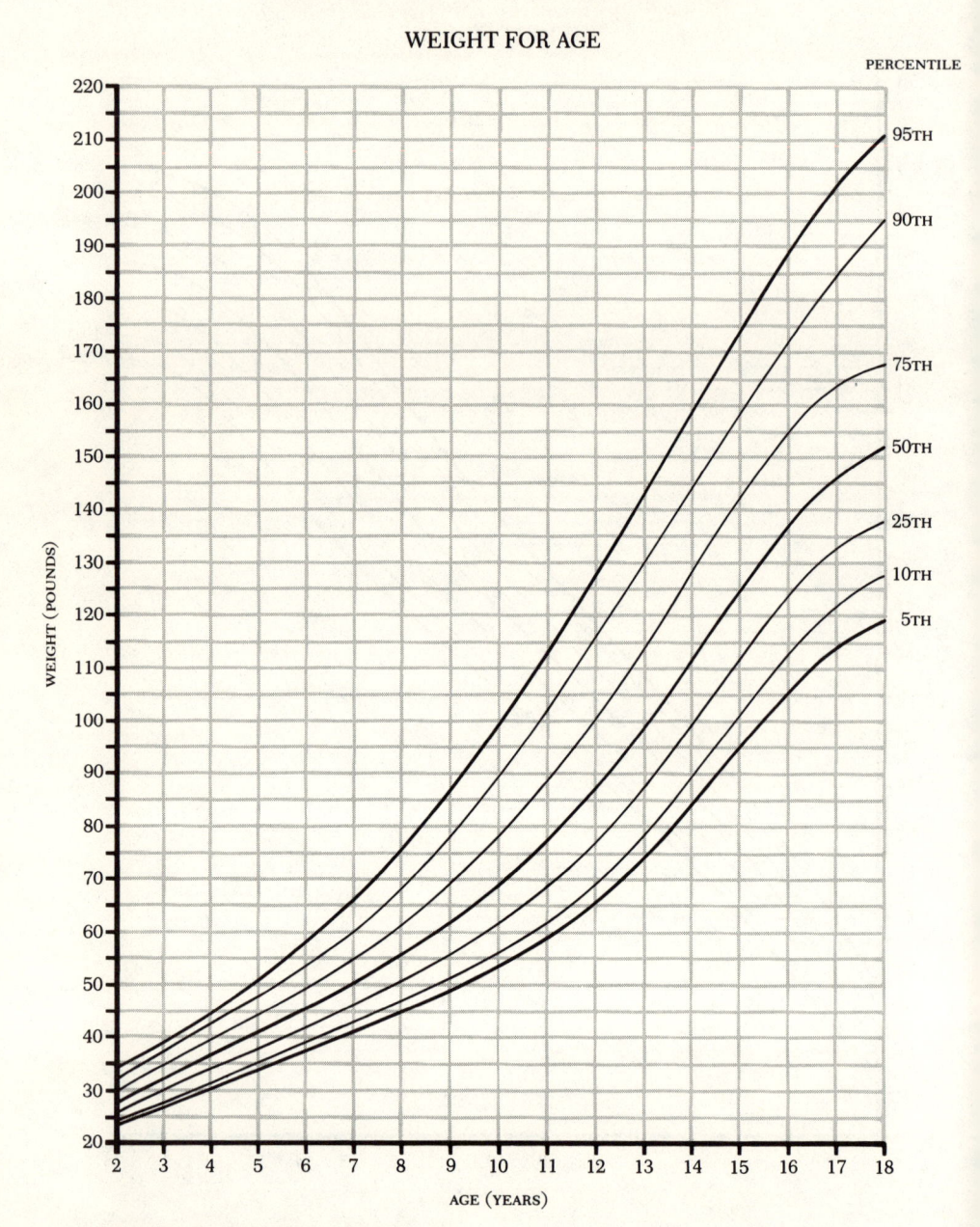

WEIGHT FOR AGE

need to lose all 40 pounds. Rather, she may have to lose only 20 to 30 pounds because by the time she is twelve and a half she should have grown an inch or two. Since many factors determine proper weight, it is important that your doctor help you set a weight goal. *Again, let me stress that you should use these growth charts only to get a very general idea of what your weight goal should be.*

Set a target date. Take the number of pounds you need to lose to reach your weight goal and divide by two (which is the average number of pounds you will lose in a week). This new number tells you how many weeks it should take you to reach your goal. Give yourself a couple of weeks' leeway and try to set the target date on a day that has some significance such as a holiday, your birthday, a family reunion, or the beginning of the new school year. Circle the date on a calendar and start thinking about how good you are going to look and feel on that day. Don't squawk because you think losing two pounds a week is too slow a pace. This is not a crash diet. You are asking for big trouble if you try to lose weight too rapidly, because the only way to drop pounds fast is to starve yourself or go on a diet that doesn't have enough essential nutrients. A crash diet is nothing more than a punishment for being overweight. Besides, most if not all of the weight lost on a crash diet is put back on. Keep in mind that while you are dieting, you must still maintain your health. The best way to do that is to develop a new eating pattern as you lose weight steadily—and slowly.

Start a personal journal. Buy a notebook, scrapbook, album, or diary to record your progress during the diet. You will use this journal to jot down your weight and body measurements, write letters to yourself, and keep photographs of yourself, as I'll explain in the next few pages. Your words and pictures will show how much thinner you are getting as the weeks roll by and how your actions, attitudes, and health are gradually improving. Don't be afraid to write down your true feelings or to include unflattering photos, since you don't have to let anyone else see your journal.

Write letters to yourself. Before you begin the diet, write a letter to yourself in your journal, describing how you feel. Mention any hassles you have at school or with friends or relatives because of your weight problem. Write down your hopes and fears and any other feelings about dieting. Then at least once a month, write yourself a new letter. Answer questions such as, "How do I feel about my body now?" "What good things have happened to me in the past month?" "How many ways have I changed?" "How do I feel physically and emotionally?" These letters will help you get to know yourself better.

Take photographs of yourself. On the day before you start the diet, have someone you trust take a few photographs of you. First, get into a T-shirt and shorts and be photographed from the front, side, and rear. Then hop into an outfit you wear often (even if the buttons are straining and the seams are splitting) and be photographed from the front. Mark on the back of each photo your weight and the date. Then, every month, be photographed in your T-shirt and shorts from the front, side, and rear. Keep those photos in your journal and look at them every month. When you look back at the way you were, you will have proof positive that you are getting slimmer and slimmer. Once you reach your goal, put on the outfit that you were photographed in at the beginning of the diet, and be photographed once again. What a difference!

Take body measurements. To follow your body's progress on the diet, measure yourself weekly and record the results in your journal. Use a cloth tape measure to figure out how big you are around your chest at the nipples, around your waist at the belly button, around your hips at their widest part, and around your thighs halfway between your knees and groin. There might be a week or two when you haven't lost any weight, yet you've lost some flab around your waist. That's okay because if your measurement is less than the week before, you are getting rid of fat.

Get a good scale. If possible, buy a new one so you know for sure that it is accurate. Don't keep it in the bathroom because moisture in the room will rust it and make the readings unreliable. Put the scale on a hard, level surface (not on carpet) in your room or in the closet and leave it there. If you keep moving it around, it won't read true. Once you start the diet, weigh yourself without any clothes on once a week—no more, no less. Do this in the morning before breakfast each week at the same time and on the same scale. Record your weight in your journal every week. Don't hop on the scale every three hours or even every day, because your weight tends to fluctuate throughout the day by as much as three pounds and that could drive you crazy. And don't try weighing yourself on other scales because they will probably give you different readings. Remember, your weight is your business—no one else's.

Bawl yourself out. When you are really looking bad—so bad that a Peeping Tom would gag—head for the mirror and give yourself a good tongue-lashing. Blast yourself for every physical fault you can find. Call yourself every rotten name in the book. Get all of this verbal poison out of your system because once you have finished raking yourself over the coals, that is it. No more attacks. No more raps at the way you look. No more whipping yourself. This diet has no room for self-pity. From now on, after your one-time-only self-roasting, you face the mirror every day and say, "I'm looking better . . . I like myself . . . I can do it!" Mean every word of it, too.

Sharpen your appearance. Some of the young people who show up at my classes for the first time look as if they came straight from the ragpickers' convention in Skuz City. They make punkers look respectable. Uncombed, greasy hair. Stained, untucked shirts. Too tight, zipper-busted skirts. Because they are fat and feeling lousy, they figure, "What's the use in cleaning up my act?" Fortunately, they usually wise up. Whether you like it or not, we are judged to some extent on our appearance. If you look like a bum, others assume you are a bum and pretty soon you end up believing it yourself. So take pride in your appearance if you haven't already. You feel much better about yourself when you improve your looks and grooming habits. You gain self-respect. So before you embark on this diet, go out and get your hair cut or styled, toss out your torn clothes, battle those zits, straighten your posture, wear clean and ironed clothes. These actions make you feel good, and with each pound you lose on the diet you begin looking better than ever.

Buy an outfit in the size you want to be when you reach your goal. It could be a skirt, blouse, pants, shirt, swimsuit, or sweater. Keep it where you can see it as a constant reminder of what you will be able to wear soon. Some of the girls in my classes bought miniskirts and hung them on their closet doors with a handwritten sign saying, "I can do it!" It's the first thing they see when they wake up in the morning and the last thing they see when they go to bed at night.

Get physical. Make up your mind that you are going to be more physically active. It doesn't have to be anything drastic. Don't think you must do lots of calisthenics. However, you can if you want. Devote a half-hour a day, four or more times per week, to some form of continuous physical activity such as aerobics, jazzercise, jogging, walking, swimming, dancing, or skating. If you can burn off 250 extra calories a day this way, you lose an extra two pounds per month. A half-hour's worth of nonstop swimming uses up 360 calories; dancing, about 325 calories; fast walking, 300 calories. If you take a fast thirty-minute walk every day for a month, you will use up 9,000 calories—good for more than two pounds a month.

If you want to exercise in a gym or health spa, terrific. Exercise that tones muscles may not reduce your weight but it can trim your measurements slightly.

Do whatever activity appeals to you. Join the activities at your local Y, join a youth group, or try out for intramural sports at school. Don't complain that sports are too hard or that you aren't good at them or that you don't have the time. These excuses helped get you fat in the first place. These excuses helped prepare you for a lifetime of watching rather than doing. Look for ways to squeeze more physical activity into each day. Walk or ride a bicycle instead of riding in a car or on a bus. Climb stairs instead of taking elevators. Walk the dog instead of letting your little brother do it.

It's absolutely essential that you get into the habit of being physically active. You benefit in several ways: You lose weight faster and more easily. You spend less time thinking about, or eating, food. You have fun. You feel better mentally. You reduce stress, tension, and fatigue.

Hold a family meeting. After reading the book, but before you start the diet, sit down with your parents and other members of the family to discuss the diet with them. Seek their support and understanding. Tell them that you have the determination and discipline needed to succeed and that with their cooperation, the challenge of reaching your goal will become much easier. Seek agreement on how much or how little you plan to tell them about your progress. If you have a good relationship with your parents, then perhaps you may want to keep them fully informed. If you confide in your parents, they can give you support and encouragement. They can also be there to listen when the going gets a little tough for you. But if you are uncomfortable with such an arrangement, then explain your feelings. Perhaps you believe that dieting is a very personal thing and the less said about it the better. Whatever arrangement you think can help the most, tell your parents. By establishing the ground rules before you start your diet, you can save yourself and your parents a lot of needless hassles later.

By the time you finish all the preparations for the diet, you are psyched up and ready to take on one of the biggest challenges of your life so far. You are ready to embark on the road to slimness.

6

THE DIET

When young people first look at the foods and guidelines of the You Can Do It! Kids Diet, they are delighted because it's all so simple. And they are somewhat disappointed because it's all so simple. They had been led to believe that in order to lose weight you need to go on some gimmicky lose-weight-quick scheme. Or some all-you-can-eat-of-the-food-you-hate plan. Or the starve-yourself-to-death-to-live-better approach.

What you really need is a no-nonsense, back-to-basics eating plan. And that's what this diet is. On it, you eat an average of 1,400 to 1,500 calories a day of common kinds of food. You eat three tasty, filling, nutritious meals a day. You eat foods low in fats and calories and high in energy and carbohydrates. This diet is chock-full of a variety of foods and drinks. That's good news not only for your taste buds but for your body as well, because these foods offer a wide range of necessary nutrients. As you know, you must take care of what's inside your body if you are going to improve the outside. You may find that some of your favorite foods are not on the diet—these foods helped make you fat. Other foods that you may not have liked in the past are on the diet. But when you give them a chance, you should end up acquiring a taste for them.

Before you review the diet in detail, keep in mind that what you eat on this plan is not diet food. It is healthy food. Eaten in the right way and in the proper amounts, it will help you lose weight steadily, safely, and gradually. This eating plan has worked for thousands of young people. It will work for you too.

What You Can Eat

MAIN CHOICES FOR BREAKFAST

1 serving of unsweetened, fortified, or enriched ready-to-eat cereal such as

Cheerios	Puffed Rice
Corn Chex	Rice Krispies
cornflakes	shredded wheat
40% Bran Flakes	Team
Grape-Nuts	Total
Life	Wheaties

OR

1 serving cooked fortified or enriched grain cereal such as

farina
oatmeal

OR

1 egg (no more than three times a week) with 1 slice whole wheat toast

MAIN CHOICES FOR LUNCH OR DINNER

3 ounces of any of the following high-fat meats (no more than three portions of high-fat meat a week)

    hamburger   roast beef
    liver   steak
    pork chops

    OR

3 ounces of any of the following low-fat meats

    lean lamb
    veal

    OR

3 ounces of any of the following poultry choices (skinless white meat only)

    chicken
    Cornish hen
    turkey

    OR

2 franks made of either turkey or chicken (no more than once a week)

    OR

3 ounces of any of the following seafood

    bass   catfish
    butterfish   clams
    carp   cod

crabmeat
dolphin (not the
    porpoise, the fish)
flounder
haddock
halibut
kingfish
lobster

oysters
pike
pompano
salmon
shrimp (7 medium-sized)
trout
tuna (water-packed)

OR

2 ounces of any of the following cheeses (no more than three portions of cheese a week)

American
Cheddar
Monterey
mozzarella

Muenster
provolone
Swiss

OR

½ cup of any of the following cheeses (no more than three portions of cheese a week)

low-fat cottage cheese (3% milkfat or less)
farmer's cheese
ricotta cheese
pot cheese

VEGETABLES

3 to 4 cups a day of any combination of the following fresh or frozen vegetables

asparagus
bean sprouts

beets
bok choi

broccoli
Brussels sprouts
cabbage
carrots
cauliflower
cucumber
eggplant
green beans
greens (beet, chard,
    dandelion, kale,
    mustard, turnip)
green peppers

mushrooms
okra
onions
red peppers
rhubarb
rutabaga
sauerkraut (washed)
spinach
summer squash
tomato
zucchini

AND

1 medium baked potato (no more than twice a week)

AND

As much as you want of the following

celery
chicory
endive
escarole

lettuce
parsley
radishes
watercress

FRUITS

3 portions a day of any of the following

1 medium apple
½ cup unsweetened
    applesauce
3 medium fresh apricots
1 small banana (no more
    than 3 a week)

½ cup blackberries
½ cup blueberries
¼ small cantaloupe
10 large cherries
½ medium grapefruit
12 large grapes

2-inch wedge honeydew melon
½ small mango
1 medium nectarine
1 medium orange
1 medium peach
1 medium pear
½ cup pineapple
2 medium plums
2 medium prunes
¾ cup raspberries
12 large strawberries
1 large tangerine
1 cup watermelon

OR

In place of 1 fruit portion, 4 ounces of any of the following

unsweetened apple juice
unsweetened grapefruit juice
unsweetened orange juice
unsweetened pineapple juice

BREADS

1 medium pita bread (also known as pocket bread) each day

OR

2 slices whole wheat bread each day (plus an additional slice when eating an egg for breakfast)

BEVERAGES

1 quart (32 ounces) of liquid each day of such drinks as

unsweetened apple, grapefruit, orange, or pineapple juice (4 ounces, in place of 1 fruit portion)
seltzer with lemon or lime
sugar-free, caffeine-free soda (no more than one a day)

decaffeinated coffee
tea (no more than 2 cups of caffeinated tea a day)
mineral water
water

AND

three 8-ounce glasses of low-fat milk each day

OR

In place of 1 milk serving:

1 cup low-fat, plain, unflavored yogurt

SEASONINGS AND SWEETENERS

Moderate amounts of the following

- allspice
- bay leaves
- basil
- chives
- cinnamon
- curry powder
- dill
- dried onion flakes
- dried garlic
- dry mustard
- Equal (or other nonsaccharin, noncaloric sweetener)
- extracts
- fresh garlic
- garlic powder
- ginger
- Italian herb seasoning
- lemon juice
- lime juice
- mint
- mustard
- nutmeg
- oregano
- paprika
- parsley
- pepper
- rosemary
- sage
- salt (as little as possible)
- tarragon
- thyme
- vinegar

FATS

No more than 2 teaspoons of reduced-calorie margarine a day
No more than 3 tablespoons of mayonnaise a week
No more than 3 tablespoons of reduced-calorie, noncreamy salad dressing a day

SNACK

1 cup popped popcorn a day

Here are the guidelines to follow:

You must weigh and measure your food. An inexpensive dietetic food scale, obtained at a health food store or drugstore, will help you determine the proper amount of food to eat. Weigh food *after* it is boned, trimmed, and cooked. Meat, fish, and poultry shrink when cooked. For example, a four ounce raw hamburger weighs three ounces when it's cooked.

You should have a complete set of measuring cups and spoons. Don't rely on table silverware spoons or coffee cups to measure. Here is the standard table of weights and measurements:

```
 3 teaspoons        = 1 tablespoon
16 tablespoons      = 1 cup
 1 cup              = 8 ounces or ½ pint
16 ounces           = 1 pound
 2 cups             = 1 pint
 2 pints or 4 cups  = 1 quart or 32 ounces
 4 quarts           = 1 gallon
```

Eat three complete meals a day. Your meals must include a main choice as well as the other food items called for in the diet. If by some unavoidable circumstance you do miss a meal, you can't make up for it by eating more at the next meal. Otherwise, before you know it, you will end up eating one giant meal—and that's no way to lose weight. Breakfast is important, so don't miss it. You say you have to catch the school bus at 7:00 A.M. and there's no time for breakfast? Get up fifteen minutes earlier. If you aren't willing to find the time, then you are not ready for this diet. Breakfast is no big production. How hard is it to pour a bowl of cereal and eat a piece of fruit? Breakfast gives you important nutrients that you need to start the day. Make the time for breakfast even if it's just you and the cat in the kitchen while everyone else is sleeping. (In many households, the early riser gets the bathroom all to himself and doesn't have to worry about the others using up all the hot water.)

Eat whole-grain, fortified or enriched, unsweetened breakfast cereals. Although they may contain some salt and sugar, the benefits far outweigh the disadvantages. First, they provide carbohydrates. Second, they are high in fiber content. Third, there is such a wide variety of cereals to choose from that breakfast should be more enjoyable for you. Avoid instant hot cereals because they are loaded with sodium. Buy regular hot cereals instead. Use fruit to sweeten the cereal. To determine how much cereal to eat, check the box label for the amount of one serving.

Eat no more than three eggs per week. Eggs are excellent sources of protein but the jury is still out on whether or not eggs contain too much cholesterol, a fatty substance that circulates in the bloodstream. If you have an egg for breakfast, you should eat one slice of whole wheat toast or half a pita so that you have consumed enough fiber for the day.

Many young people in my classes say they poach or hard boil an egg rather than scramble or soft boil it because there is more to sink their teeth into when it's cooked that way. You can have an egg any style, but if you fry it, use a nonstick fry pan or a spray-on vegetable coating. You can also use a teaspoon of soft, reduced-calorie margarine. (But remember, it counts as one of the two teaspoons of reduced-calorie margarine that you are allowed per day.)

Eat cheese no more than three times a week. Cheese is a good source of calcium and protein, but some are relatively high in salt and fat.

Eat no more than three portions of high-fat meat per week. Beef and pork are good sources of protein and minerals. However, even when trimmed, beef and pork contain fat and that is why you must limit your consumption of these meats. For the same reason, do not eat beef or pork franks. Other meat, fish, and poultry on the diet can be eaten every day but make sure all visible fat is cut off before you cook it. Make sure you peel off the skin of chicken, turkey, or Cornish hen because it's loaded with fat. Eat only the white meat, which is lower in calories than dark meat.

Your foods can be braised, broiled, boiled, roasted, charcoal-grilled, steamed, or stewed. They can also be cooked in a microwave, a wok (an Oriental cooking pan), a nonstick fry pan, or SilverStone pans. Fruits and vegetables can be eaten raw, of course.

You must eat 3 to 4 cups of vegetables per day. They should be fresh or frozen only, because canned or processed vegetables are laced with salt and chemicals. If you are one who doesn't include vegetables on your list of One

Hundred Favorite Foods, then here's some straight talk: Vegetables have been getting a bum rap for too long. Too often they are the last items to be eaten, or are shoved over to one side of the plate. Give them a chance. Surely there have been foods that you disliked at first but grew to enjoy. The same will happen with vegetables. Since they come in all shapes, sizes, colors, textures, and flavors, there are bound to be some that you will like. You might as well try them. You really don't have much of a choice if you want to stick to this diet, because vegetables play a crucial role in helping you slim down. Because of their high fiber content, they fill you up without skyrocketing your calorie count. And because most of them are crunchy, it takes you longer to eat them. That means they are more satisfying than some food you can gobble down in two bites.

Many people agree that raw or lightly cooked vegetables taste better than fully cooked ones. Overcooking them destroys nutrients and can turn them into bland mush. Vegetables should be washed thoroughly, and are especially good when served with various seasonings. In addition to eating them raw, young people enjoy vegetables that are steamed or cooked in a wok, both of which leave the vegetables slightly crunchy. In addition to 3 to 4 cups of vegetables a day, you are allowed to eat 2 medium-size baked potatoes (plus skins) a week.

Feel free to eat one or two salads a day. You can eat as much as you want of lettuce, chicory, endive, escarole, parsley, radishes, and watercress in your salads. If you wish, include a portion of your vegetables in the salad. You can use 3 tablespoons of low-calorie salad dressing per day, but avoid all creamy dressings because they are higher in fats and calories.

Eat three portions of fresh fruit every day. You can train your sweet tooth to accept fruit the way it used to crave candy. Use one of your fruits to sweeten your breakfast cereal or to make a fruit shake before bedtime. Eat your fruits throughout the day—with meals or as snacks—to help you maintain a good energy level. You may eat canned fruit only if it is unsweetened and in its own juice. For one of your daily portions of fruit, you may substitute a 4-ounce glass of unsweetened fruit juice. Most people would rather eat the fruit than drink juice because fruit, with its high fiber content, is more filling and lets you gnaw on something. It only takes a few seconds to gulp down juice, compared to a few minutes to eat a piece of fruit.

You should eat one whole piece of medium-sized pita bread per day. It's much better than regular bread because it's chewy and therefore takes longer to eat. You can stuff lettuce, sliced raw vegetables, and other goodies into the pita without worrying about food falling out of your sandwich. As a substitute, you can eat two slices of whole wheat bread (but somehow sandwiches won't seem as much fun). Whatever bread you choose, make sure it is either enriched or fortified, which means it has been strengthened with vitamins and minerals that had been lost during processing.

Drink three 8-ounce glasses of low-fat milk every day. Stay away from whole milk because it contains too much fat. Your best choice is acidophilus milk, a kind of low-fat milk sold in most cities throughout the country. It's sweeter than regular milk and contains a bacteria culture, thermophilic acidophilus, which is thought to make the milk easier to digest. If you aren't thrilled about drinking milk plain, then use it on your breakfast cereal or make milkshakes (see the recipes in chapter 9). If you are allergic to milk, then have one cup of low-fat, unsweetened, plain yogurt three times a day. You can mix the yogurt with fresh fruit or cereal.

Drink at least 32 ounces (1 quart) of liquid per day in addition to milk. Water is by far the best beverage you can drink because it quenches your thirst and contains no calories. You can have mineral water, seltzer, or plain water flavored with lime or lemon juice. It's okay to drink decaffeinated coffee and herbal teas, but drink no more than two cups of regular tea per day because it contains caffeine. Don't gulp a lot of fluids before or during your meal. It could fill you up so much that you won't eat all your food. That's not good because an hour or two later you will become famished and end up eating more than you should.

If you absolutely, positively must have a soda, then have a 12-ounce can of sugar-free, caffeine-free soda. But no more than one per day. Don't drink soda during your meal. Otherwise the carbonation bloats your stomach and gives you a false sense of feeling full. As a result, you eat less, but then a short time after your meal, when the bloating subsides, you feel hungry and may end up eating too much.

Feel free to season your food. Too much salt is harmful, as you already know, so use as little as possible. Try to spruce up the taste of your foods with other seasonings listed on the diet.

You can also use small amounts of vegetables (such as a slice or two of onion or ¼ cup of chopped tomato) as a flavoring in your meal preparation without counting them in your day's vegetable allotment.

You can use artificial sweeteners—as long as they are noncaloric and nonsaccharin. A natural, safe sweetener is Equal, one of a growing number of NutraSweet products. However, I suggest you limit your use of sweeteners because they only encourage you to retain a taste for highly sweetened foods. By gradually reducing the amount of sweetener used, you teach your taste buds to prefer naturally sweet food.

Limit your use of fats. Have no more than two teaspoons of reduced-calorie margarine a day. It's best to use soft margarine in a tub because it's much easier to spread and you are less likely to use too much. Spray-on vegetable coating can be used when cooking.

For an evening snack you can have one cup of popped popcorn. But skip the salt and butter. The best way to pop popcorn is in a microwave or in a hot air popper. Popcorn goes great with a milkshake and is quite filling (besides providing you with fiber and other nutrients).

There is no need to buy dietetic food. Most special diet foods are expensive and many are not much lower in calories than regular foods.

Do not buy any diet pills or appetite suppressants. They are only crutches and serve no useful purpose to you because you are learning a new way of eating.

As you can see, this diet has no gimmicks, no tricks. It's simple common sense. If you are looking for an easy way to lose weight, then stop reading and give this book away. If you want to diet, then diet right. To make yourself look better, you must eat better. And with the right attitude, you can make adjusting to this diet easier on yourself.

7

FOURTEEN-DAY SAMPLE MENU

Forget the food that you used to eat. Don't concentrate on what you can't have. The surest way to fall off the diet is to think about "forbidden foods." Instead, go into this diet thinking about all the foods you *can* eat and all the new foods you are going to try. It's a new eating experience. You are going to learn what green beans taste like without three pats of butter and four shakes of salt; what a baked potato tastes like without a mound of sour cream and artificial bacon bits; what cereal tastes like with strawberries instead of three heaping spoonfuls of sugar.

To lose weight, you must simply follow the diet. You may think that by the time you reach your goal you will be the color of a broccoli spear and your head will be shaped like a zucchini. But what will really happen is that you will end up enjoying basic foods.

The foods on this diet can be combined to make satisfying, filling meals. Take a look at the fourteen-day sample menu.

Note: If a dish listed in this sample menu section is made from a recipe in this book, it will say "see recipe." Please consult Index for page numbers. Also, to determine how much cereal to eat, check box label for the amount of one serving.

DAY 1 **Thursday**

BREAKFAST

1 serving shredded wheat
1 cup acidophilus low-fat milk
1 medium peach, sliced

LUNCH

1 chicken salad sandwich made with
    3 ounces skinless cooked chicken breast, diced
    ¼ cup chopped celery
    1 tablespoon mayonnaise
    ½ cup shredded lettuce
    1 medium pita bread
1 medium raw carrot, cut into sticks
1 medium orange
Beverage

DINNER

3 ounces roast beef, lean only
½ cup Seasoned Mushrooms (see recipe)
1 cup cooked fresh or frozen green beans, with
    1 teaspoon reduced-calorie soft margarine
2 cups tossed garden salad, with
    2 tablespoons reduced-calorie salad dressing
1 cup acidophilus low-fat milk

SNACK

1 cup popped popcorn
1 Piña Colada Milkshake (see recipe)

DAY 2 **Friday**

BREAKFAST

1 large egg, any style
1 slice whole wheat toast, with
    1 teaspoon reduced-calorie soft margarine
½ medium fresh grapefruit
1 cup acidophilus low-fat milk

LUNCH

1 roast beef sandwich made with
    3 ounces sliced roast beef, lean only
    1 tablespoon mayonnaise
    ½ medium tomato, sliced
    lettuce
    1 medium pita bread
½ medium cucumber, cut into spears
1 medium apple
Beverage

DINNER

3 ounces baked skinless chicken breast
1 medium baked potato, with
    1 teaspoon reduced-calorie soft margarine
1 cup cooked fresh or frozen broccoli, with
    1 squirt fresh lemon juice
2 cups tossed garden salad, with
    2 tablespoons reduced-calorie salad dressing
1 serving Frozen Banana Chips (see recipe)
1 cup acidophilus low-fat milk

SNACK

1 cup popped popcorn
1 Coffee Milkshake (see recipe)

DAY 3 **Saturday**

BREAKFAST

1 serving 40% Bran Flakes
1 cup acidophilus low-fat milk
½ cup fresh blueberries

LUNCH

1 Pita Bread Cheese and Mushroom Pizza (see recipe)
1 stalk celery, cut into sticks
12 large Frozen Grapes (see recipe)
Beverage

DINNER

One 3-ounce Broiled Lamb Chop, lean only (see recipe)
1 cup cooked fresh or frozen cauliflower, with
    1 teaspoon reduced-calorie soft margarine
1 cup fresh or frozen cooked spinach, with
    1 teaspoon reduced-calorie soft margarine
2 cups tossed garden salad, with
    2 tablespoons reduced-calorie salad dressing
¼ small cantaloupe
1 cup acidophilus low-fat milk

SNACK

1 cup popped popcorn
1 peppermint milkshake (see Milkshake Marvel recipe)

DAY 4 *Sunday*

BREAKFAST

2 slices Whole Wheat French Toast (see recipe), with
    1 serving Cinnamon-Margarine Topping (see recipe)
1 medium tangerine
1 cup acidophilus low-fat milk

LUNCH

2 medium turkey franks, with
    ½ teaspoon mustard
½ cup washed sauerkraut
1 medium pear
Beverage

DINNER

3 ounces Broiled Fish Fillet (see recipe)
1 cup Green and Red Pepper Combo (see recipe)
1 cup fresh or frozen asparagus, with
    1 teaspoon reduced-calorie soft margarine
2 cups tossed garden salad, with
    2 tablespoons reduced-calorie salad dressing
1 cup watermelon cubes
1 cup acidophilus low-fat milk

SNACK

1 cup popped popcorn
1 Chocolate Milkshake (see recipe)

DAY 5 **Monday**

BREAKFAST

⅔ cup cooked enriched farina
1 cup acidophilus low-fat milk
1 small banana

LUNCH

1 cheese sandwich made with
    2 ounces Swiss cheese
    lettuce
    ½ teaspoon mustard
    1 medium pita bread
1 medium raw carrot, cut into sticks
12 large fresh strawberries
Beverage

DINNER

1 serving Burger Romano (see recipe)
1 cup cooked fresh summer squash, with
    1 teaspoon reduced-calorie soft margarine
1 cup fresh or frozen Brussels sprouts, with
    1 teaspoon reduced-calorie soft margarine
2 cups tossed garden salad, with
    2 tablespoons reduced-calorie salad dressing
1 cup acidophilus low-fat milk

SNACK

1 cup popped popcorn
1 peach milkshake (see Fruity Milkshake recipe)

DAY 6 *Tuesday*

BREAKFAST

1 large egg, any style
1 slice whole wheat toast, with
    1 teaspoon reduced-calorie soft margarine
1 medium orange
1 cup acidophilus low-fat milk

LUNCH

1 tuna salad sandwich, made with
    3 ounces canned water-packed tuna, drained
    ¼ cup chopped celery
    1 tablespoon mayonnaise
    ½ cup shredded lettuce
    1 medium pita bread
½ medium cucumber, cut into spears
2 medium plums
Beverage

DINNER

1 serving Roast Chicken-in-a-Pan Dinner (see recipe)
1 cup cooked fresh or frozen green beans, with
    1 teaspoon reduced-calorie soft margarine
2 cups tossed garden salad, with
    2 tablespoons reduced-calorie salad dressing
1 serving Cinnamon Apple Slices (see recipe)
1 cup acidophilus low-fat milk

SNACK

1 cup popped popcorn
1 vanilla milkshake (see Milkshake Marvel recipe)

DAY 7 Wednesday

BREAKFAST

1 cup oatmeal, with a dash of cinnamon
1 cup acidophilus low-fat milk
One 2-inch wedge honeydew melon

LUNCH

1 cheese hoagie made with
    2 ounces mozzarella cheese
    ½ medium tomato, sliced
    ½ cup shredded lettuce
    1 tablespoon reduced-calorie Italian salad dressing
    1 medium pita bread
1 celery stalk, cut into sticks
10 large cherries
Beverage

DINNER

3 ounces roast veal, lean only
1 cup Zucchini and Carrots (see recipe)
1 cup mashed turnips with
    1 teaspoon reduced-calorie soft margarine
Tomato and Cucumber Salad (see recipe)
1 cup acidophilus low-fat milk

SNACK

1 cup popped popcorn
1 banana milkshake (see Fruity Milkshake recipe)

DAY 8 Thursday

BREAKFAST

1 large egg, any style
½ medium pita bread, toasted, with
    1 teaspoon reduced-calorie soft margarine
4 ounces unsweetened grapefruit juice
1 cup acidophilus low-fat milk

LUNCH

1 chicken sandwich made with
    3 ounces skinless cooked chicken breast, sliced
    1 tablespoon mayonnaise
    ¼ cup raw bean sprouts
    ½ cup shredded lettuce
    1 medium pita bread
½ cup raw broccoli
1 large tangerine
Beverage

DINNER

One 3-ounce broiled pork chop
1 medium baked potato, with
    1 teaspoon reduced-calorie soft margarine
1 cup cooked bok choi
2 cups tossed garden salad, with
    2 tablespoons reduced-calorie salad dressing
½ cup unsweetened applesauce
1 cup acidophilus low-fat milk

SNACK

1 cup popped popcorn
1 Coffee Milkshake (see recipe)

DAY 9 *Friday*

BREAKFAST

1 serving Rice Krispies
1 cup acidophilus low-fat milk
12 large fresh strawberries

LUNCH

1 shredded-Cheddar cheese sandwich made with
    2 ounces shredded Cheddar cheese
    ¼ cup sliced fresh mushrooms
    ½ cup shredded lettuce
    1 tablespoon reduced-calorie Catalina salad dressing
    1 medium pita bread
1 celery stalk, cut into sticks
12 large grapes
Beverage

DINNER

1 serving Skewered Shrimp (see recipe)
1 cup cooked fresh or frozen spinach, with
    1 teaspoon reduced-calorie soft margarine
1 cup cooked fresh beets, with
    1 teaspoon reduced-calorie soft margarine
1 medium tomato, cut into wedges, with
    1 tablespoon reduced-calorie salad dressing
1 cup Fruity Yogurt (see recipe)
Beverage

SNACK

1 cup popped popcorn
1 Chocolate Milkshake (see recipe)

DAY 10 *Saturday*

BREAKFAST

1 serving cornflakes
1 cup acidophilus low-fat milk
½ medium fresh grapefruit

LUNCH

2 medium chicken franks, with
    ½ teaspoon mustard
1 medium pita bread, sliced into two halves
½ medium tomato, sliced
1 small banana
Beverage

DINNER

3 ounces roast lamb, lean only
1 cup fresh or frozen asparagus, with
    1 teaspoon reduced-calorie soft margarine
1 cup cooked fresh or frozen cauliflower, with
    1 teaspoon reduced-calorie soft margarine
2 cups tossed garden salad, with
    2 tablespoons reduced-calorie salad dressing
1 cup acidophilus low-fat milk

SNACK

1 cup popped popcorn
1 pineapple milkshake (see Fruity Milkshake recipe)

DAY 11 **Sunday**

BREAKFAST

1 large egg, any style
1 slice whole wheat toast, with
    1 teaspoon reduced-calorie soft margarine
¼ small cantaloupe
1 cup acidophilus low-fat milk

LUNCH

1 Cottage Cheese Salad OR Vegetable Salad and Dip OR Vegetable-Cheese Dip (see recipes)
1 cup watermelon cubes
Beverage

DINNER

1 hamburger made with
    3 ounces cooked lean ground beef
    1 medium slice onion
    ½ medium tomato, sliced
    2 lettuce leaves
    ½ teaspoon mustard
    1 medium pita bread
1 cup cooked fresh or frozen green beans, with
    1 teaspoon reduced-calorie soft margarine
1 celery stalk, cut into sticks
1 cup acidophilus low-fat milk

SNACK

1 cup popped popcorn
1 raspberry milkshake (see Fruity Milkshake recipe)

DAY 12 **Monday**

BREAKFAST

1 serving Cheerios
1 cup acidophilus low-fat milk
½ cup fresh blueberries

LUNCH

1 tuna salad sandwich made with
    3 ounces canned water-packed tuna, drained
    ¼ cup chopped celery
    ½ cup shredded lettuce
    1 tablespoon mayonnaise
    1 medium pita bread
½ medium cucumber, cut into spears
1 medium orange
Beverage

DINNER

3 ounces skinless roast turkey breast
1 medium baked potato, with
    1 teaspoon reduced-calorie soft margarine
1 cup cooked fresh or frozen broccoli, with
    1 teaspoon reduced-calorie soft margarine
2 cups tossed garden salad, with
    2 tablespoons reduced-calorie salad dressing
1 serving Chocolate Turtles (see recipe)
1 cup acidophilus low-fat milk

SNACK

1 cup popped popcorn
1 almond milkshake (see Milkshake Marvel recipe)

DAY 13 *Tuesday*

BREAKFAST

1 Pepper and Onion Scramble (see recipe)
1 slice whole wheat toast, with
    1 teaspoon reduced-calorie soft margarine
3 fresh medium apricots
1 cup acidophilus low-fat milk

LUNCH

1 turkey sandwich made with
    3 ounces skinless roast turkey breast
    1 tablespoon mayonnaise
    ½ medium tomato, sliced
    ½ cup shredded lettuce
    1 medium pita bread
6 radishes
1 large tangerine
Beverage

DINNER

3 ounces broiled steak, lean only
½ cup Seasoned Mushrooms (see recipe)
1 cup cooked fresh summer squash, with
    1 teaspoon reduced-calorie soft margarine
1 Broiled Tomato Italiano (see recipe)
2 cups tossed garden salad, with
    2 tablespoons reduced-calorie salad dressing
1 cup acidophilus low-fat milk

SNACK

1 cup popped popcorn
1 strawberry milkshake (see Fruity Milkshake recipe)

DAY 14 **Wednesday**

BREAKFAST

1 serving Total
1 cup acidophilus low-fat milk
2-inch wedge honeydew melon

LUNCH

1 cheese and onion sandwich made with
    2 ounces American cheese
    ¼ cup sliced onions
    ¼ cup shredded lettuce
    ½ teaspoon mustard
    1 medium pita bread
1 stalk celery, cut into sticks
10 large cherries
Beverage

DINNER

3 ounces Cornish Hen (see recipe)
1 cup cooked fresh or frozen carrots, with
    1 teaspoon reduced-calorie soft margarine
2 cups tossed garden salad, with
    2 tablespoons reduced-calorie salad dressing
1 cup acidophilus low-fat milk

SNACK

1 cup popped popcorn
1 Sunshine Orange Milkshake (see recipe)

You may have noticed three things about this diet:

The diet starts on a Thursday. That's a great day to begin a diet. Almost everyone starts diets on a Monday, which is the worst day of the week. Think about it: You just get over a fun weekend and now you have to face school. What a drag. Imagine adding the responsibility of a new diet. Your body and mind just aren't geared up to get off to a good start on a Monday. However, by Thursday the week is almost over and you are filled with the happy anticipation of the coming weekend. Your body and mind are revved up and ready to tackle the new dieting challenge.

You get to eat more than you thought possible on a reducing diet. Most plans are much more restrictive, which makes it much more uncomfortable to diet. This means that the chances of a dieter quitting increase dramatically. On the You Can Do It! Kids Diet, you eat enough so you are not hungry, you lose weight gradually so you have a better chance of keeping it off, and you develop good eating patterns.

The meals seem so plain. They are plain. This diet is not going to pamper you or trick you with imitation low-calorie substitutes or hide the real taste of foods under sauces and gravies. Plain food is good food. And for a change, you get to find out how good plain, basic foods taste. They are marvelous.

A final word about the foods on this diet: Don't compare them with what you have been shoveling into your mouth in the past. It's a whole new ball game. For example, you can make fruity milkshakes, but don't think for a moment that these taste as thick and creamy as the milkshake at Dairy Queen. It's not meant to be an imitation. You can't compare low-cal food with high-cal food. It's like trying to compare a pickup with a Corvette. They are meant for different things. The food on this diet is meant to give you nutrients as it helps you lose weight. High-cal junk food does nothing more than taste good. Let's take another example: pita bread pizza. Delicious. But no way does it taste like a pizza with loads of cheese dripping off the sides. Once you are on the diet, you acquire new tastes and eat things you swore you would never touch. These foods please your taste buds and help make you thin. The choice is yours. Do you want to wolf down six slices of greasy, thick-crusted pizza-parlor pizza with a pitcher of soda and waddle away from the table like an overstuffed teddy bear? Or do you want to enjoy the new tastes of a homemade pita bread pizza and a fruity shake, feeling satisfied in your stomach and your heart that you are eating right and losing weight?

8

TAKING CHARGE

There is one ingredient you won't find on any sample menu, but it is essential to success on this diet. The ingredient is responsibility.

You must take charge. You can't always depend on Dad to tell you what to eat. You can't expect Mom to do all the shopping and food preparation. You can't always rely on your friends to keep you from temptation. This is your challenge, and it's your duty to make this diet work. You and you alone are responsible for everything you put in your mouth. This responsibility begins even before you pick up a knife and fork. It starts with planning your menus, assisting with the grocery shopping, making sure the right kinds of food are available in your home, and helping prepare the meals.

Creating Menus

After studying the diet and sample menus, you now know what you can eat. The next step is to make out your own weekly menu. To do this, write down all the allowed foods that you like and those that you are willing to try. Plan your meals for the week around these foods, making sure you have included the necessary required foods and have met all the other guidelines on the diet.

For starters, you might want to follow the fourteen-day sample menu until you become more familiar with the diet. Then go ahead and be adventurous. Each week, change the menu by choosing new foods on the list. There is enough variety on this diet for you to be able to prepare many different kinds of meals. Don't be afraid to experiment in the kitchen (as long as you choose allowed foods).

Restricted foods should be spaced evenly throughout the week. For example, since you can have two baked potatoes per week, you might plan to eat a baked potato on Monday and another on Thursday. If you eat them on consecutive days, then you must wait six days before you can have another one. By spacing out restricted foods that you like, you always have something extra special to look forward to. To help you keep track of restricted foods, make a chart that you can run off on a copy machine. On the left side of the chart, list the foods and the number of times you are allowed to eat them in a week. Then as you eat these foods, make a check mark.

> *Rick, twelve, 15 pounds overweight:* When I first started doing my menus, I ate my three portions of [high-fat] meat and two baked potatoes during the first two days on the diet. Boy, did I have a tough time the rest of the week because all I ate for a main course after that was chicken—and I got pretty sick of that. Now when I plan the menu, I make sure I have something I really like every day.
>
> *Julie, thirteen, 25 pounds overweight:* At first I stuck to the sample menus because I thought that was the easiest thing to do. The real reason, though, was because I was part lazy

and part afraid. After a month, I got bored eating the same things so I forced myself to make up menus. Each week I try one new food on the diet. Sometimes the new food isn't bad at all, like asparagus. Sometimes the food is the pits, like Brussels sprouts.

When you are planning the weekly menu, talk it over with whoever does the grocery shopping in your household. Try to coordinate your meals so that you eat many of the same basic foods as the rest of the family. This saves money at the grocery store as well as time and effort preparing meals. Also, think of ways you can use leftovers when planning your menus. If you are having broiled chicken for dinner, plan on making a chicken salad sandwich for lunch the next day. And plan your meals around fruits and vegetables that are in season, because that's when they are usually at their lowest prices.

Grocery Shopping

After you write out your weekly menu, prepare a grocery list of the items you need and help with the shopping. Because the diet stresses fresh fruits and vegetables, some of which may spoil if kept around too long, you may have to make two runs to the store every week.

Once in the supermarket, pick out only those items that you have on your grocery list and choose the brands that appeal to you. Take advantage of coupons and special sales only if those foods are on the diet.

To make shopping a little easier, many young people make up a list of all the foods they like and need on the diet. They run this list off on a copy machine. Then every week they take one of the lists and mark what they want for the week and use it to do the shopping. (It's also handy when you can't get to the store. Just mark off the things you need, and whoever shops for the family can pick up those items for you.)

"But wait," you say. "Won't I be tempted if I grocery shop?" Unless you walk in blindfolded and wear nose plugs, chances are you can be tempted, especially if you are hungry. So don't you dare go to the grocery store on an empty stomach, because you might buy everything in sight. Eat one of your fruits before you shop, or go to the supermarket only after you have eaten a full meal. That should help. But it's all up to you. Whether it's the grocery store or the dining room table or the school cafeteria, you are going to be faced with temptation daily until you get into a healthy eating pattern. You can't avoid it. You must learn to deal with it.

If you have a problem with temptation, then make yourself a deal: Reward yourself with a nonfood treat every time you purchase only those foods that are on the diet. This reward could be something like bath oil or a new magazine. Believe it or not, young people on this diet who really believe in themselves, who really succeed, aren't fazed by the grocery store test of temptation. They pick up their pita bread right next to the bakery section. They walk past the potato chips to get to the produce bins. (I have more to say about temptation in later chapters.)

> *Darrel, eleven, 22 pounds overweight:* When I go food shopping, I only go down aisles that have my food. I don't go out of my way to be tempted. But a lot of times there's an open box of cookies at the bakery counter that they want customers to sample. I just walk on by.

> *Eva, fifteen, 28 pounds overweight:* I do the shopping for the whole family. That way I can make sure I'm getting the foods that I want and need for the diet. I let Mom relax and read her book on the bench outside the store while I grocery shop. I enjoy doing it.

Suzanne, fourteen, 34 pounds overweight: I buy all fresh fruits and vegetables at a small stand near my house because it's cheaper and better. I told the owner his produce stand was helping to make me slim. Now he always asks about my progress on the diet and he sells me fruits and vegetables at a special lower price.

Planning Ahead

The food on the diet must be available in your house. You don't want to run short of certain necessary foods and end up eating something you shouldn't as a substitute. *Plan ahead.* Have enough of the right kinds of food for several days in advance.

Double-check the next day's menu. For example, if you want a scrambled egg, an orange, and whole wheat toast for breakfast on Wednesday, check the refrigerator Tuesday to make sure you have the items. You don't want to wake up and say, "Darn, no eggs or bread, so I guess I'll have some frozen waffles." It's also wise to make your school lunch the night before and keep it in the refrigerator (or else have the ingredients ready for the morning). Besides, it saves time if you are a late sleeper or a slow starter in the morning. The important thing is to have the food available. Your success is based on the food that is in your home. You can't say, "Well, I've been following the diet this week, but now that we're out of tuna, I'll just have to buy my lunch at school because there's nothing here to fix." That's a sure way to fall off the diet.

A strange thing often happens when you buy certain foods for yourself that no one in the family cares about eating. They suddenly develop a craving for them. Let's say you like apples. You buy seven for the week so you can have one every day. But by the third day they are gone because your family is now on an apple kick. What do you

TAKING CHARGE 103

do? Either buy more apples or tell the family "hands off." Some dieters have a special place in the refrigerator, kitchen cabinet, or pantry that is just for their food and can't be eaten by the rest of the family. There's nothing wrong in saying politely, "That's my food. Please leave it alone." If you are eating your one cup of popcorn as an evening snack, don't let the others in your family have any of your portion. Make some for them or let them pop their own. That might put you in a position of appearing selfish. But you must stick to your guns. It's your food and your diet. You are not being selfish. It's just that you are dedicated to losing weight and the rest of the family must understand that.

> *Luis, fifteen, 26 pounds overweight:* If someone in my family tries to eat from my stash of food for the diet, I say, "I want to be thin and I know you want me to lose weight too, so please don't take my food or ask for a bite."
>
> *Craig, twelve, 21 pounds overweight:* I have a large plastic bin in the refrigerator and I keep all my fruits, salad fixings, and vegetables in it. I also taped my name on it. It works because nobody in the family tries to rip off any of my food.
>
> *Sarah, fourteen, 31 pounds overweight:* There is nothing worse than going to the fruit bowl for that last apple and seeing your father eating it. That happened to me a couple of times, so I decided to use colored stickers. I put little bright green round stickers right on my apples, bananas, and oranges so that the rest of the family knows those fruits are off limits to them.
>
> *Matt, thirteen, 28 pounds overweight:* I have a section of the pantry that is all mine. I have a weekly checklist on the door and when I take out any food, I check it off the list. That way I always know what is there and when I go grocery shopping I know exactly what I need to get.

Preparing Meals

You can't always expect to relax in front of the TV or listen to your favorite records in your room while someone else is preparing your meals. You must pitch in. Even if you don't know the difference between a grater and a colander, there are still many things you can do to help make your meals. If your mother does the cooking, ask her what you can do to help. You can make the salad; slice, dice, or chop the vegetables; peel the skin off the chicken; cut the fat off the pork chop; and lots of other things.

Remember, you must weigh and measure your food (after it is trimmed and cooked). No, you aren't going to have to weigh food for the rest of your life. Quite the contrary. After a few weeks of using the food scale, you will develop a sense of how much things weigh just by looking at and holding them. Eventually, you won't need to weigh anything. Even if you are an old hand in the kitchen and know how to cook, I still want you to use a food scale for a few weeks at least.

> *Kay, seventeen, 33 pounds overweight:* I didn't get a food scale at first because I thought I knew how much everything weighed by feel. I was wrong. After a month on the diet, I borrowed a friend's food scale and found that I was cheating myself out of about one ounce of meat and chicken with every meal.

If you aren't involved in some phase of your meal preparation, then you leave yourself open to trouble. It's too easy for others to be careless if they are preparing your meals. For example, while fixing dinner, your sister may decide to substitute creamed corn, which is not on the diet, for the green beans on your menu. The more you can do to help prepare your meals, the better off you will be.

Terri, fourteen, 33 pounds overweight: I prepare parts of my meals on Sunday afternoon when the rest of the family is watching football on TV. I clean all my fresh vegetables and chop them or slice them. I put the vegetables and things for my salads in a large, airtight, plastic covered bowl, which keeps everything fresh for up to four days. When I need something, it's all there ready for me to use.

Julie, thirteen, 25 pounds overweight: On Saturdays I start making my weekday meals. I have a bunch of frozen dinner trays. I fill them with chicken or meat and vegetables and cover them with foil and pop them into the freezer. When it gets near supper time during the week, I take one of the frozen dinners out and heat it up.

Marianne, fifteen, 30 pounds overweight: I like to cook so now I make the whole family's meals. Because I am in charge of the kitchen, I plan their meals around my menu. They're eating healthier now and I eat the things that are good for me. All of us feel better without junk foods. Best of all, I don't have any dull chores—my sister has to do them all because I do the cooking. With me in charge of the kitchen, Mom gets a break because she's so tired when she comes home from work.

To take the fullest advantage of this diet, I recommend that you have on hand a steamer, a blender, and a nonstick frying pan.

The steamer is a handy device that holds vegetables above the water so that they can be steamed in a covered pot. Steaming retains more nutrients than other forms of cooking do.

The blender is especially good for making milkshakes and whipping up a scrambled egg. As you experiment with meals on the diet, you can find many other uses for it. If your blender cannot chop ice finely, I suggest you buy an ice crusher to make your milkshakes.

By using a nonstick pan, such as SilverStone, you can fry an egg or make French toast and other foods with a small amount of low-calorie margarine—or without any at all.

Here are some other preparation tips:

- ✔ Clean all your vegetables at one time so they are ready when you need them.
- ✔ If you can't use all your fresh vegetables before they get too ripe, put them in sealed plastic bags and freeze them or share them with the rest of the family.
- ✔ Cook as many foods ahead of time as you can. Then when you need them, take them out of the freezer and put them into boiling water or in the microwave.
- ✔ Instead of freezing a whole pound of hamburger meat, make individual four-ounce patties (which shrink to three ounces when cooked) and freeze them until you are ready to use them.
- ✔ Buy lean bottom round roast and ask the butcher to grind it. Ground round has less fat then regular ground beef.
- ✔ When taking a salad to school for lunch, put your salad dressing in a separate container and pour the dressing on the salad when you are ready to eat.

If helping to prepare foods is going to be a new experience for you, don't be overwhelmed by all the suggestions and guidelines in this chapter. The tips are pretty basic. Nobody is going to expect you to be a master chef. Do as much as you feel comfortable with. But remember, you are responsible for the food you eat.

9
RECIPES

Fixing complicated meals is no fun when you're dieting, so the recipes in this book are quick and easy to prepare. I can remember going to weight reduction classes when I was fat and being handed pages of recipes. Nine times out of ten, the recipes were not only difficult to make but also hard to swallow. The dishes weren't as great as the diet counselor had promised and they certainly didn't taste anything like I thought they would. After not eating what I'd spend hours cooking (maybe that was the diet plan: fix things you can't eat) and looking at the kitchen counter crowded with dirty bowls, spoons, and pots, I'd become so frustrated that I'd decide to eat something else—something convenient and fattening.

You have enough other things to do without also having to worry about cooking elaborate meals. When you finish preparing the recipes in this book, you'll have plenty of time left over for extracurricular activities, homework, chores, and just plain relaxation.

Breakfast Dishes

PEPPER AND ONION SCRAMBLE

vegetable cooking spray
2 tablespoons sliced red onions
2 tablespoons sliced green pepper
1 large egg
1 tablespoon low-fat milk

Apply a thin coat of vegetable spray to a small nonstick frying pan. Sauté the sliced onion and green pepper over medium heat, stirring frequently. Cook for about 5 minutes, or until the onion and green pepper are slightly crunchy. In a small bowl, combine the egg with the milk and beat well. Gather the onion and green pepper mixture in the center of the frying pan. Reduce heat to low. Pour the beaten egg mixture on top of the onion and green pepper. Quickly mix together, stirring frequently, until the egg is cooked.

WHOLE WHEAT FRENCH TOAST

1 large egg
2 tablespoons low-fat milk
½ teaspoon vanilla extract
2 slices whole wheat bread

In a shallow bowl, beat the egg well. Stir in the milk and vanilla extract. Soak the bread slices in the egg mixture. Cook over medium heat in a nonstick frying pan until the bread slices are golden brown on both sides. While the

French toast is cooking, prepare the Cinnamon-Margarine Topping (see following recipe).

CINNAMON-MARGARINE FRENCH TOAST TOPPING

1 teaspoon reduced-calorie soft margarine
2 teaspoons water
1/8 teaspoon cinnamon
Dash of nutmeg
1 packet Equal

Stir all ingredients together in a very small saucepan over low heat until the margarine is completely melted. Keep warm until French toast has finished cooking. Top French toast with the mixture.

Salads

TOMATO AND CUCUMBER SALAD

1 medium tomato, sliced
1/2 medium cucumber, sliced
Dash of oregano
1 tablespoon reduced-calorie salad dressing

In a small bowl, combine tomato and cucumber slices, oregano, and salad dressing. Toss gently, cover tightly, and place in the refrigerator to marinate for about 15 minutes. This makes one flavorful serving of salad that adds zest to any dinner.

COTTAGE CHEESE SALAD

½ cup shredded lettuce
½ cup low-fat cottage cheese
¼ cup chopped scallions
¼ cup chopped celery
½ medium raw carrot, shredded
½ medium cucumber, sliced
½ medium green pepper, sliced
2 tablespoons reduced-calorie Catalina salad dressing

Place the shredded lettuce on a large salad plate. Spoon the cottage cheese on top of the lettuce in the center of the plate. Arrange the chopped scallions, chopped celery, shredded carrot, and cucumber and green pepper slices around the cottage cheese. Pour the salad dressing over the salad.

VEGETABLE SALAD AND DIP

½ cup low-fat cottage cheese
1 tablespoon finely chopped green pepper
1 medium raw carrot, grated
1 tablespoon finely chopped onion
1 tablespoon low-fat milk
Assorted raw vegetables

In a small bowl, combine the cottage cheese, green pepper, carrot, onion, and milk. Mix well. Store in the refrigerator until you're ready to use it. This makes a delicious dip for raw vegetables such as broccoli, cauliflower, cucumber, carrots, celery, and green peppers.

Main Dishes

CORNISH HEN

    1 Cornish hen
    ¼ teaspoon tarragon
    ¼ teaspoon parsley
    One 6-ounce can orange juice concentrate, thawed

Preheat oven to 350°F. Split the hen in half, wash it, and pat it dry with paper towels. Sprinkle it with the tarragon and parsley and rub them in with your fingers. Place it on a broiler pan and bake in the preheated oven for 1 hour and 15 minutes. Baste with the orange juice every 15 minutes while the hen is baking. Make sure to eat only 3 ounces of white meat.

BROILED LAMB CHOP

    One 4-ounce lamb chop, weighed after it is trimmed
        of bone and fat
    ½ teaspoon freshly ground pepper
    ½ teaspoon oregano
    1 garlic clove, minced
    2 teaspoons lemon juice
    1 tablespoon mustard
    Vegetable cooking spray

In a small, shallow baking dish, combine all the ingredients except the lamb chop and the cooking spray. Dip the chop into the mixture. Be sure to coat it well on both sides. Marinate the chop in the mixture in the refrigerator for 2 hours, turning and basting occasionally. Remove the chop and place it on a broiler pan that has been coated with vegetable cooking spray. Broil for 5 minutes. Turn the chop over and brush with the leftover marinade. Broil for an additional 5 minutes.

SKEWERED SHRIMP

7 medium shrimp, fresh or frozen
6 whole bay leaves
1 large green pepper, cut into 1-inch squares
½ cup fresh pineapple chunks
¼ fresh lemon

Thaw the shrimp if they are frozen. On 2 thin metal skewers, alternate the shrimp, bay leaves, green pepper squares, and pineapple chunks. Place the skewers on a broiler pan and broil for 3 minutes. Turn the skewers over, squeeze the juice from the lemon over the shrimp, and broil for an additional 2 minutes. Remove from the heat and discard the bay leaves. This is extra delicious when cooked outside on a charcoal grill.

BROILED FISH FILLET

4 ounces fresh fish fillet
Vegetable cooking spray
¼ teaspoon paprika
¼ fresh lemon

Wash the fish and pat it dry with paper towels. Place the fish on a small cookie sheet or broiler pan that has been coated with a vegetable cooking spray. Sprinkle the paprika on top of the fish. Broil for approximately 5 minutes. Squeeze juice from the lemon over it and broil for an additional minute or so. The fish is done when it flakes easily with a fork.

VEGETABLE-CHEESE DIP

>2 ounces Cheddar cheese, grated
>2 tablespoons low-fat milk
>Assorted raw vegetables
>Dash of pepper

In a small pan, combine and mix the cheese and milk over a low heat. Stir constantly. Pour the mixture into a dish. Season with pepper. Dip raw vegetables such as broccoli, cauliflower, cucumber, carrots, celery, and green peppers into the heated cheese.

PITA BREAD CHEESE AND MUSHROOM PIZZA

>1 medium pita bread
>2 slices fresh tomato
>½ cup sliced fresh mushrooms
>2 ounces mozzarella cheese, sliced
>Garlic powder
>Italian herb seasoning or oregano

Split the pita bread open into two round halves. Lay the halves cut side up on a foil-covered cookie sheet. Place a slice of tomato on each half. Arrange ¼ cup of mushrooms on each half. Place 2 ounces of cheese on top of the tomato slices and mushrooms. Sprinkle garlic powder and Italian herb seasoning or oregano on top of the cheese, as desired. Broil until the cheese melts and turns light brown.

ROAST CHICKEN-IN-A-PAN DINNER

1 large chicken breast, skinless
1 medium potato, washed, peeled, and quartered
½ cup chopped celery
Dash of salt
Dash of pepper
Dash of tarragon
1 to 1½ cups water
1 cup sliced carrots

Preheat oven to 350°F. Wash the chicken breast and place it bone side up in an 8-by-8-inch baking pan. Arrange the potato and chopped celery around the chicken. Season with a dash of salt, pepper, and tarragon. Add one cup of water. Bake in preheated oven for 30 minutes. Turn chicken over and add the carrots. Cook for 30 additional minutes. Add ½ cup of water if mixture looks too dry.

BURGER ROMANO

4 ounces lean ground chuck, made into a
    hamburger patty
⅓ cup chopped onion
⅓ cup chopped green pepper
½ cup finely chopped tomato
⅛ teaspoon garlic powder
¼ teaspoon Italian herb seasoning or oregano
¼ cup water

In a small skillet, brown the hamburger patty over high heat approximately 2 minutes on each side. Remove from heat. Drain the hamburger patty on paper towels. Pour off the grease and wipe the pan clean. Combine the remaining ingredients in the pan with the water. Place the browned hamburger patty on top of the mixture. Bring to a boil, cover, and reduce heat to a simmer. Cook for 10 to 15 minutes. Check occasionally, spooning the vegetable mixture over the hamburger. Add a little more water if it looks too dry. Serve with the vegetables on top of the hamburger patty.

Vegetable Side Dishes

SEASONED MUSHROOMS

1 pound fresh mushrooms
2 tablespoons water
Dash of garlic powder

Wash the mushrooms well. Sometimes they are very dirty and you must rub each one to get it clean. Dry them thoroughly. Slice the mushrooms lengthwise if small, or into several pieces if large. Place the mushrooms in a large nonstick frying pan with the water. Sprinkle with garlic powder according to your taste. Cover the pan and cook over a medium high heat until the mixture starts to boil. Reduce heat to low, and continue to cook for an additional 5 minutes. The mushrooms will have produced a lot of broth that is terrific over steak and hamburger. This recipe makes approximately 2 cups. Remember to eat only the serving portion that you are allowed. Share the rest with your family or store it in the refrigerator and reheat it the next day.

BROILED TOMATO ITALIANO

1 medium tomato
Dash of garlic powder
Dash of Italian herb seasoning or oregano
Dash of pepper

Wash the tomato and cut out its core. Slice it in half. Place the tomato cut side up on a foil-covered cookie sheet, and sprinkle it with garlic powder, Italian herb seasoning or oregano, and pepper. Broil 10 to 12 minutes about 8 inches away from the flame or heating coils until the tomato is hot and juicy.

GREEN AND RED PEPPER COMBO

1 medium green pepper
1 medium red pepper
1 small onion, sliced
1 small clove garlic, sliced
¼ teaspoon dill weed
1 tablespoon water

Wash the peppers thoroughly and cut them in half. Remove all the seeds and pulp. Slice the peppers in long strips approximately 1 inch wide. In a small skillet, combine the onion, garlic, dill weed, and water. Cover and steam the mixture for 3 minutes. Add the green and red pepper slices and cook, covered, approximately 5 minutes, or until the peppers are slightly tender. Watch to make sure that the water does not boil away. You may have to add a little water while the peppers are cooking. Drain the vegetables, discard the garlic, and serve hot.

ZUCCHINI AND CARROTS

2 medium carrots
1 medium zucchini
¼ teaspoon dill weed
¾ cup water

Scrub and peel the carrots and cut off their ends. Scrub the zucchini. Slice the zucchini and carrots in quarters lengthwise. Place the carrots and water in a skillet with a lid. Cook, covered, over medium heat for 7 to 10 minutes or until they are slightly tender. Add the sliced zucchini and dill weed. Cover and cook 3 additional minutes until the zucchini sticks are slightly tender. Drain and serve.

Desserts

CHOCOLATE TURTLES

⅓ cup unsweetened canned pineapple chunks, in their own juice
1 tablespoon unsweetened pineapple juice
1½ teaspoons Swiss Miss chocolate flavor mix sweetened with NutraSweet

Drain the juice from the pineapple chunks, reserving the juice in a separate container for later use. In a very small cup or bowl, mix one tablespoon of the pineapple juice with the chocolate flavor mix until it is well blended. Dip each pineapple chunk into the mixture, rolling it around until it is well coated. Place the chunks on a foil-covered cookie sheet. Freeze for at least 4 hours.

CINNAMON APPLE SLICES

1 medium apple
3 tablespoons water
Dash of cinnamon
1 packet Equal

Peel the apple. Cut it into quarters and remove its core. Then cut the apple into thin slices. Place the slices in a small nonstick frying pan with the water. Sprinkle with cinnamon. Cover the pan and place over high heat until the mixture comes to a boil. Reduce the heat to low and cook an additional 5 minutes, or until the apple slices are tender. Remove from heat and stir in the Equal.

Here's a tip: Once in a while, for a special treat, sprinkle the cooked Cinnamon Apple Slices with a teaspoon of Grape-Nuts cereal.

FROZEN GRAPES

12 large seedless grapes

Wash and dry the grapes. Place them on a piece of foil. Freeze for at least 4 hours. Eat them while they are still frozen.

Here's a tip: If you freeze grapes in the morning, they will be ready to eat when it's time for your last fruit of the day.

FRUITY YOGURT

12 large fresh strawberries
1 cup plain low-fat yogurt
1 to 2 packets Equal

Wash, stem, and slice the strawberries. In a salad or soup bowl, stir the yogurt and Equal together thoroughly. Then gently fold in the sliced strawberries.

Here's a tip: You can substitute any of the fruits on the diet for the strawberries. Favorites are blueberries, peaches, and bananas.

FROZEN BANANA CHIPS

- 1½ teaspoons Swiss Miss chocolate flavor mix sweetened with NutraSweet
- 1 tablespoon low-fat milk
- 1 small banana
- 1 tablespoon Grape-Nuts cereal

In a small bowl, combine the chocolate flavor mix with the milk. Stir until the mixture is smooth and creamy. Cut the banana into ½-inch chunks. Dip each banana chunk into the chocolate mixture until well coated, then place on a foil-covered cookie sheet. Sprinkle the chocolate-covered banana chunks with the Grape-Nuts. Freeze for at least 4 hours.

Milkshakes

PIÑA COLADA MILKSHAKE

½ cup unsweetened canned pineapple chunks, in their own juice
1 cup low-fat milk
1 to 3 packets Equal
¼ teaspoon vanilla extract
¼ teaspoon coconut extract
4 ice cubes, crushed

Drain the juice from the pineapple chunks, reserving the juice in a separate container for later use. In a blender, combine the pineapple chunks, milk, Equal, and vanilla and coconut extracts. Add 2 tablespoons of the reserved pineapple juice. (Store the rest of the juice in the refrigerator for other shakes, to make chocolate turtles, or to drink as a fruit juice.) Add the crushed ice cubes. If you do not have an ice crusher, you can place the cubes directly into a blender if it can chop up ice finely. Cover and blend on high speed for about 60 seconds. The recipe makes approximately 2 cups of a delicious, thick milkshake.

COFFEE MILKSHAKE

1 cup low-fat milk
1 to 3 packets Equal
¼ teaspoon vanilla extract
1 teaspoon decaffeinated instant coffee
4 ice cubes, crushed

In a blender, combine the milk, Equal, vanilla extract, and coffee. Add the crushed ice cubes. Cover and blend on high speed for about 60 seconds. Makes approximately 2 cups of a rich and creamy shake.

FRUITY MILKSHAKE

    1 cup low-fat milk
    1 to 3 packets Equal
    ¼ teaspoon vanilla extract
    One of the following fruits:
        12 large fresh strawberries
        ½ cup unsweetened canned pineapple, in its own juice
        ½ cup fresh blueberries
        ¾ cup fresh raspberries
        1 small banana
        1 medium peach, peeled and sliced
    4 ice cubes, crushed

In a blender, combine the milk, Equal, vanilla extract, and one of the fruit choices. Add the crushed ice cubes. Cover and blend on high speed for about 60 seconds. This makes approximately 2 cups of a rich and creamy shake. There are many fruity taste-tempting milkshakes for you to create.

MILKSHAKE MARVEL

    1 cup low-fat milk
    1 to 3 packets Equal
    ¼ teaspoon vanilla extract
    ¼ teaspoon vanilla (additional), almond, peppermint, or coconut extract
    4 ice cubes, crushed

In a blender, combine the milk, Equal, vanilla extract, and one of the extract choices. Add the crushed ice cubes. Cover and blend on high speed for about 60 seconds. This makes approximately 2 cups of a zesty shake. If you have already used up your fruits for the day, or if you prefer eating your fruits separately, then a Milkshake Marvel is right for you.

CHOCOLATE MILKSHAKE

1 cup low-fat milk
2 teaspoons Swiss Miss chocolate flavor mix
   sweetened with NutraSweet
4 ice cubes, crushed

In a blender, combine the milk with the chocolate flavor mix. Add the crushed ice cubes. Cover and blend at high speed for about 60 seconds. This makes about 2 cups of a velvety smooth chocolate delight.

SUNSHINE ORANGE MILKSHAKE

1 cup low-fat milk
1 to 3 packets Equal
¼ teaspoon vanilla extract
4 ounces unsweetened orange juice
4 ice cubes, crushed

In a blender, combine the milk, Equal, vanilla extract, and orange juice. Add the crushed ice cubes. Cover and blend at high speed for about 60 seconds. This makes approximately 2 cups of a frothy milkshake.

10

THE GOOD EATING HABIT

There is more to this diet than just eating the right foods. It is just as important to learn when, where, and how to eat. In other words, you must develop good eating habits.

As I mentioned in chapter 3, "Why You Are Fat," you weren't born with bad eating habits. You learned them. Now you are going to unlearn them. Otherwise, eating the right foods won't necessarily mean you will lose weight. So before you start the diet, make up your mind to change those bad eating habits. After all, they helped make you fat.

Bad eating habits are not hard to correct. In just a few short weeks you can unlearn them and learn good ones that you can follow for the rest of your life. You know some of them already, such as eating three meals a day, substituting fresh fruits for sweets, and reducing the portions of your meals. But there are several other important good eating habits to follow.

Chew your food slowly. You don't have to sit there and count to ten every time you put a forkful of food in your mouth. But you should take several seconds to chew food, leaving it in your mouth for as long as you feel comfortable. Savor the taste, feel the texture, enjoy the aroma. For instance, instead of gobbling up an orange in thirty seconds flat, invest a few minutes in it. First, peel it slowly and catch a few whiffs of the scent. Feel the thick orange skin. Now slowly bite into one section at a time, letting the flavor linger on your tongue. Now that's the way to enjoy a snack.

Sip, don't gulp your drinks. A couple of gulps and your beverage is already in your stomach and you are ready for more. Try sipping your drink and give your taste buds a chance to enjoy the flavor.

Make each meal last at least twenty minutes. If you finish your meal in under ten minutes, congratulations. You could win a gold medal—if speed eating ever becomes an Olympic event. Since that's not likely to occur in the next century, there's no reason to shovel food into your mouth at the speed of light. Come up for air between bites, wipe your mouth with your napkin, carry on a conversation with others at the table. To help extend the time of the meal, cut your food into small pieces and eat them one at a time. Also, put one kind of food in your mouth at a time, instead of spearing a few green beans and a piece of chicken simultaneously.

Kevin, twelve, 24 pounds overweight: Eating too fast was a problem for me. To slow down, I decided to talk more at the dinner table. Now, throughout the day when I learn interesting things, especially in school, I remember to talk about them at dinner. The more I talk, the longer it takes for me to eat. My parents say dinner is more pleasant because I have lots of interesting things to talk about.

Andre, fourteen, 26 pounds overweight: I play classical music on the radio when we sit down to eat and that seems to slow me down. I'm not crazy about the music but my parents like it.

Alex, fourteen, 27 pounds overweight: I used to finish ahead of everyone else at supper because my brothers and sisters are slowpokes. Now I watch the way they eat and I've slowed down, because you tend to eat the same way other people at the table eat. I look at people instead of looking down at my plate all the time.

Peter, fourteen, 46 pounds overweight. All I have to do is think of Uncle Charlie and I slow down. I used to love food as much as my uncle, but when I went on my diet, I saw how disgusting it looks to eat so fast. Now I can't stand being at the same table with him. The other day he was wolfing down a meatball sandwich. His chin was greasy from the gravy and he kept stuffing that sandwich in his big mouth and trying to talk at the same time. It was gross.

Eat only in the dining room or kitchen. Let either of these rooms become the "eating" room. This should help you cut down on any unnecessary eating, especially snacking in front of the TV or in your bedroom.

Stop eating when you are full. That means you must resign from the clean plate club. You should not have to finish everything on your plate if you are full. You are not a human garbage can. If there is food on your plate that you have not touched, put it away as a leftover or, as a last resort, give it to the dog. It's better to waste the food than to fatten your body. Don't fall for the line, "What about the poor starving children in Africa?" You cannot help the starving people by eating everything on your plate any more than you can hurt them by throwing away the leftovers. The only person who will suffer will be you if you eat when you aren't hungry. Certainly you should try to avoid wasting food. If you find that you are leaving food on your plate regularly, then simply cut back on the size of your portions and *stop* when you are full.

Serve food restaurant style rather than family style. With a little cooperation from your family, all of you can make a slight adjustment in the way food is served at home. Have your mother put the food on the plates in the kitchen and then bring the plates to the dinner table rather than placing bowls and platters of food on the table for the family members to help themselves. By serving restaurant style, you aren't as tempted to eat second helpings or to finish off that one last piece of meat on the platter. Out of sight, out of mind.

Snack only when you are hungry. Most snacking is unnecessary. We tend to snack out of boredom, nervousness, depression, or other emotional needs. Remember what I told you about the difference between hunger and appetite? The next time you are about to reach for something to snack on, stop and ask yourself, "Am I really hungry?" If so, then help yourself to a piece of fruit or a raw vegetable or some other treat allowed on the diet. But if you yearn for a snack because you are upset or bored, then find another outlet. Go in your room, close the door, and punch the pillow and scream. Run around the block. Confide in your best friend. Read. Write a letter. Do something other than snacking.

Drink only a small amount with your meal. You and your body are entitled to consume full meals on this diet, so there is no sense in filling up your stomach with too much liquid when you are eating.

Reward yourself with nonfood treats. For instance, if you have aced a final exam, don't reward yourself with food.

What's wrong with giving yourself a nonfood treat? Save the money you would have spent on junk food and buy something for yourself: baseball cards, a ticket to see a new movie, makeup, a new football.

Keep junk food out of sight in the house. Mountain climbers scale a mountain because "it's there." Fat people eat food because "it's there." If candy and peanuts and other forbidden foods are within easy reach throughout the house, put them in the cupboard out of sight (or better yet, see if the family will give them up).

Don't sample food while cooking. You can pick up many extra calories by working in the kitchen helping with dinner. Nibbling on an end cut from a roast or sampling the family's casserole are sure ways to add unnecessary calories. To avoid temptation, help prepare the parts of the meal that are low in calories—make the salad, steam the vegetables, pour the drinks.

As an aid to learning good eating habits, some experts cite tips such as using a smaller plate so it looks as if you are eating a larger portion of food, putting down your knife and fork between each bite to slow down your eating, counting to twenty before swallowing each bite, or dressing up your plate with garnishes. These are merely tricks, which I don't encourage. You have to be honest with yourself. You know the score. This diet may not be the easiest, but if you stick with it, you will lose weight. It requires dedication and determination—especially during those important first two weeks.

11

THE FIRST TWO WEEKS

The first two weeks on the diet could be among the toughest days you ever face, physically and mentally. Yet they could also be the most rewarding.

During this time you may be riding an emotional roller coaster, eating new foods in a new way, resisting temptation, ending old habits, maybe experiencing slight headaches and stomachaches, feeling guilt, hope, nervousness, and happiness. But then you will reach a point when you feel so much better—and weigh so much less.

Here is what could happen to you during the first two weeks:

If you are like many of the young people in my classes, the night before you begin the diet, you gorge yourself on what I call "the last supper." You binge on fattening foods with second helpings at dinner and dessert, followed by late-night snacks. I can understand why you do it. You want one last fling with all those "wonderful" foods not on the diet—foods so wonderful they made you fat. "The last supper" does nothing more than reinforce your old way of eating while weakening your determination to give the new diet a chance.

Look at it this way: Imagine that you have just graduated from junior high school and you feel sad because you are going to miss some of your younger classmates and perhaps a favorite teacher. The only way you could have stayed longer in junior high was to flunk. It's time to move on to a new school and new challenges to better yourself. This diet presents a similar situation. Think of it as graduating from the old school of junk food and fattening food to a new school of healthy eating.

You're not going to ease your way into the diet. You go in all the way at once. It's no different from testing the cold water of a lake or pool. You stick your toe in, wade in up to your ankles, then up to your knees. That just makes it agonizing. It's best to jump in, get the initial shock over with, and then enjoy the refreshing water. Jump into the diet, get over the initial shock, and get on with shedding pounds.

The first day on the diet is often a breeze for "last supper" participants because their stomachs are still full from the night before. But the second day sometimes gets a little more difficult. Some young people report that they get minor headaches or stomachaches. If this happens to you, don't fret. Your body is complaining, craving for all those sweets and other nonhealthy goodies. It makes sense that your body may rebel because it's used to living on junk. It's like a spoiled child who no longer gets all the toys he wants, so he throws a temper tantrum. Likewise, your body wants that junk food and fattening food, so it throws a temper tantrum in the form of headaches and stomachaches. But within a few days it accepts—and eventually insists on—only healthy food. In a way, minor headaches and stomachaches are good signs. They mean your body is trying to adjust to a new and better way of eating. Hang in there. These symptoms last for a very short time.

Now just because I mentioned these possible brief side effects, don't tell yourself you are going to get them. I'm just warning you that *some* young people have felt this discomfort, but they managed to cope easily enough. So can you.

Marsha, sixteen, lost 20 pounds and was 32 pounds from her goal: The first day on the diet was great. I was still full from the previous day's pig-out. But on the second day of the diet I had a headache because I missed having my big handful of cookies that I always ate. After the third day I felt much better.

Bob, fifteen, lost 15 pounds and was 25 pounds from his goal: The first couple of weeks were the hardest. On the second day of the diet I had a stomachache and felt lousy. I had been eating loads of junk food for so long that that's what my body wanted. But I knew if I gave in, I'd never lose weight. That's when I sucked it in and toughed it out.

Don't be surprised if you feel very tired and lazy and want to go to bed early during the first week. You may have a strong case of the mopes, too tired to do much of anything—even fixing popcorn for your evening snack. This feeling of tiredness (if it happens at all) doesn't last long. Once your body has accepted the fact that it's being fueled by decent, healthy food, your energy level picks up. By the end of the first week, you will become more used to the diet and any physical discomfort or symptoms should disappear.

Some young people have told me they were famished during the first week of the diet. No doubt they were eating less food than before. However, when we talked about it, we discovered that they were confusing hunger with appetite (flip back to pages 45–46 for a review on this subject.) They felt hungry because they expected to feel hungry. They were so used to eating large portions of food that when they were faced with smaller meals they assumed that they would be hungry. If you think constantly about the food you can't have during the first few days on the diet, try to understand that you probably are not hungry. It's just that you miss the habit of eating a lot of fattening foods.

You may think about food more often in the evening, when you are less active. This is a time when you probably snacked quite often before you began dieting. One of the best things to do during the first couple of weeks is to go to bed early—or at least not to stay up too late. This way you are less likely to experience a growling stomach or give in to temptation. During the day, take your mind off food by changing your routine. Visit a friend after school, get your chores out of the way, put your energies into a new hobby. *Stay busy.*

> *Brad, thirteen, lost 18 pounds and was 10 pounds from his goal:* I felt very hungry the first three days. At times I didn't think I could do it. So I sat down and tried to think it out. I had kind of the same feelings I had during the first days at summer camp. I tend to get nervous when I try something new and different and I want to eat a lot then. I realized that I wasn't really all that hungry after all, so I went outside and rode my bike and promised to give the diet a chance.

> *Lucy, fifteen, lost 33 pounds and was 29 pounds from her goal:* The first days were the worst. I had that bad habit of wanting to eat even though I wasn't hungry. That's always been my problem. I want to munch throughout the day. After the fifth day on the diet, it started becoming easier for me. You have to give yourself a few days to break your old habits. To help me through the difficult times, I crochet and that keeps my hands and mind busy. I never think of this diet as making me hungry. I think of it only as giving me hope.

Some young people feel uptight during the first few days on the diet. You may find yourself snapping at your parents and friends, having a shorter temper or less patience, arguing about doing chores, or trying to put off your homework. If this happens to you, it is just because you feel different physically as a result of all the positive changes that are happening to your body. But these feelings won't last long.

No matter what else you feel, don't get caught up in feeling sorry for yourself. Why should you feel sorry? You should feel happy. At last you are correcting a problem with a solution that works. You're ahead of the game, ahead of all the other people who have problems but no solutions. You should feel happy because you are no longer eating the foods that made you fat; the foods that made others tease you; the foods that made you feel miserable. I will be the first to admit that the right foods alone won't make you thin. I could take a dozen kids to the grocery store and load them up with all the nutritious, low-calorie foods they need to lose weight, but unless they believe in themselves, unless they are willing to work for it, they won't shed a pound.

If you want to fill your mind with thoughts, make them positive ones. You don't have any room for negative thoughts or guilt feelings. Some young people feel guilty when they start to diet beause it makes them face up to the fact that they made themselves fat. At the dinner table they are prone to say, "If I had never gotten this fat, I could eat mashed potatoes and gravy like the rest of the family." Some dieters feel jealous because they can't eat what others can eat. They say things like "It's not fair that you eat anything you want." You have no reason to feel guilty because you are now solving a problem. And you shouldn't feel jealous because what others eat is of no concern to you. Negative feelings only hurt your chances of succeeding on this diet.

Tony, fifteen, lost 16 pounds and was 22 pounds from his goal: During the first week I was cranky because I had a lot of adjusting to do. But my mood brightened when I stepped on the scale and saw how much weight I lost. This diet is far from fun, but it is something I can really live with.

Try to make your meals as pleasant as possible. Avoid conversations at the dinner table that could lead to arguments. Set aside enough time to enjoy a leisurely meal with the family. This way you are more apt to remain in a good frame of mind, which helps make coping with the diet easier, especially during the first two weeks.

Marianne, fifteen, lost 18 pounds and was 12 pounds from her goal: From day one on the diet, I decided that since I was doing something special for me—losing weight—I might as well do it right. So instead of putting my food on regular plates, I use Mom's best china. She said it was okay with her. I eat my grapes out of a crystal champagne glass, and my utensils are sterling silver. It makes my meals elegant.

Kay, seventeen, lost 12 pounds and was 21 pounds from her goal: I love candles. So when I started the diet a month ago, I asked the family if we could eat dinner by candlelight. They thought it was a great idea. It's such a nice atmosphere now at the dinner table. We seem to eat slower and we all seem much more mellow. I think it's helped me handle the diet because it makes dinner so pleasant.

The biggest thrill at the end of the first week occurs when you step on the scale and see the dramatic amount of weight you have lost. The feeling of accomplishment makes you glow with pride. Depending on how overweight you are, you could lose from 5 to 8 pounds. Now that's terrific, but don't expect to lose that much every week. Much of that lost weight is water loss, not fat loss. Then every week after that, expect to drop an average of 2 pounds. It's not healthy to lose weight too fast, so be reasonable and safe—stick with losing 1 to 3 pounds a week.

At the end of the first two weeks, notice how good you look and feel. You pay more attention to the way you look, taking special care in the clothes you wear. Your hair is washed and combed. Your face looks fresh and glowing. You walk with an extra spring in your step because you are beginning to lose that bloated feeling you had in the past. You walk with pride and confidence because you have proven to yourself that you can survive quite nicely without sweets and fatty foods and whatever other junk you used to eat. You have every right to feel proud at the end of the second week. You have only to look in the mirror or stick your thumb between your belly and the waistband of your slacks or skirt to notice you are losing weight.

Your parents and close friends may mention that they can tell the difference in you already. That ought to get you fired up. However, your initial weight loss may not be very noticeable to others. Some young people carry weight better than others do. So don't be upset if you don't hear any favorable comments at first. The scale doesn't lie. You know you are losing weight.

Many young people on the diet are so excited and happy about trying to improve themselves that they are on a natural high—humming, singing, and smiling. With this wonderful attitude, they breeze through the first two weeks on the diet. The same can happen to you.

Go ahead, pump yourself up with positive feelings. Tell yourself: "I'm going to be thin. I can do it!" You are in control of your life now. And you are determined to change yourself for the better.

Diana, fifteen, lost 20 pounds and was 12 pounds from her goal: I believed from the first day on the diet that I would be a winner. I put up with the headaches and the stomachaches during those early days because I was filled with pure determination that I was going to be thinner. Heck, I had stomachaches and headaches long before I went on the diet, so they didn't mean much to me and they went away by the end of the first week. I wonder if it had anything to do with the fact that when I stepped on the scale I saw that I lost 6 pounds. My stomach actually felt flatter. Boy, was that a great feeling. You don't have to be stuffed with food to feel happy. I feel fantastic inside and out.

Luis, fifteen, lost 18 pounds and was 8 pounds from his goal: From day one I've had no problem with this diet. I really believe that when the responsibility is placed on you, you just go out and prove to yourself and everyone else that you can do it.

12

THE REST OF THE WAY

As you enter the third week on the diet, you will begin to blossom with confidence because you have cleared the hurdle of the first two weeks. You will feel more comfortable with your new way of eating. You'll look forward to each week's weigh-in because the scale lets you know that you are getting closer and closer to your goal.

If you have a lot of weight to lose, you may think it's going to take forever to reach your goal. So set up a series of short-term goals. Let's say you need to lose fifty pounds. That could seem like an overwhelming task at first. But it doesn't appear so hard to achieve when you break it up into five mini-goals of losing ten pounds each.

When you lose the first ten pounds, give yourself a reward. Treat yourself to a movie, buy a new issue for your stamp collection, pick out a new record album. Then shoot for the next mini-goal of ten pounds. After you hit it, reward yourself again. Keep doing this until you reach the big goal. A goal is nothing more than a series of little successes, and you deserve a pat on the back for each little success. Rewards help keep you motivated. Of course, what better incentive do you need than to know that one day soon you will be slim?

As you progress on the diet and the pounds fall off, a new you emerges. Your energy levels soar and there's no stopping you because you want to show yourself—and others—all the things you can do. You begin to enjoy activities that have nothing to do with food. Before, when you went to the movies, all you thought about was how much popcorn, soda, and candy you could down in two hours. Now you go to a movie to see the film. Spending rainy days in the shopping mall no longer means stopping off for a chocolate ice cream soda with whipped cream. You're dancing, roller-skating, marching in the school band, and doing a dozen different things. You're making friends and caring more about others—and yourself.

But there could be times throughout the diet when you experience a difficult week. Perhaps some problems at school or at home get you upset enough that you don't devote the proper effort to your diet. Or perhaps you get sick, in which case your top priority is to get well (even if it means eating something not called for on the diet). Or maybe you are just tired of dieting.

When you hit a rough spot during the diet, take a few minutes to give yourself a pep talk. Tell yourself: "I can do it! I can do it! I can absolutely make it on this diet. I'm going to look great and feel great. I'm going to be slim." Believe it, don't just wish it. After a month or two on the diet, you probably won't need to give yourself a pep talk because others will be giving you loads of compliments: "Wow, you're looking terrific. We can really see a difference." Just look in the mirror for confirmation. Your waist, arms and legs are thinner. Physically, you feel better than ever. You are revved up with vitality. Your body is taking on a new shape.

However, you may not look as sharp as you want because you are still wearing your oversized clothes, which make you look like a graduate of the Charlie Chaplin School of Fashion. It's very difficult for others to notice how much weight you've lost when you are clad in baggy clothes. Unless you are rolling in money, don't go on any spending sprees until you reach your goal. Why buy expensive outfits that you can wear for only a short time before they become too big on you? It's better to alter what you have or buy some practical inexpensive clothes that will get you through the next few months. Several young people in my diet classes go to consignment shops and trade their large clothes for smaller sizes. If you don't mind wearing used clothes, it's a cheap way to own a varied wardrobe while on the diet. Wait until you reach your goal and then go out and buy new clothes for the new you.

When you step on the scale each week, you will usually be charged with enthusiasm because you have lost another few pounds. But be aware that sometimes—no matter how faithful you are to the diet—you may discover to your shock that you haven't lost an ounce that week. In fact, you may have gained. Don't scream, cry, or throw the scale through the window. You have just hit a plateau. It's nothing unusual.

A plateau is a relatively short period of time during dieting when your body does not lose weight despite your best efforts. To put it in very simple terms, the body is undergoing a dramatic readjustment and sometimes it takes a week-long breather before it responds again to your dieting efforts. You might never experience a plateau, but if you do, be patient. Simply continue to follow the diet and by the following week you should once again be losing weight. Whatever you do, don't panic.

Michael, sixteen, lost 18 pounds and was 34 pounds from his goal: I hit a week when I didn't lose any weight even though I stayed true to the diet. I couldn't believe it. I weighed myself at least ten times a day, waiting for the scale to show me that I had lost a few pounds. My being good on the diet depended on what the scale said. But when it didn't say what I wanted, I got so mad I polished off a whole bag of cookies. I know that sounds dumb but that's what happened. I have since learned that no matter what the scale says, you are going to lose weight if you stick to your guns and stay on the diet. I only weigh myself once a week, and no matter what it tells me, I stick to the diet.

Girls who are in their premenstrual phase are likely to experience a monthly plateau. Just before and during their periods, girls may feel bloated and can weigh up to three pounds more than the previous week because their body is retaining fluid. As a result, they can be heavier without being fatter. In other words, the scale is measuring weight but it can't measure fat. The extra weight from water retention disappears at the end of the menstrual period.

For some young people, the last few weeks on the diet are the hardest. Here's why: As you near your goal, your weekly weight loss may be less than what you have been averaging throughout the diet. This is because your body is adjusting to its new weight and its caloric needs may be changing. At this stage, you might lose one pound or maybe half a pound per week.

Don't feel disappointed. After all, you are still on a remarkable trend—losing weight. Stay positive. Each pound lost is a step closer to your ultimate goal. You are not in a race, so don't get hung up about how fast you can lose weight.

Some young people get so anxious to reach their goals that in desperation they starve themselves for a few days or skip meals. So what happens? They become hungry—very hungry—and eat more than they should and actually gain weight. Then there are those young people who share the same attitude as Brian.

Brian, fourteen, lost 38 pounds and was 10 pounds from his goal: I'm proud that I've made it this far but now I lose one pound a week at most. Sometimes I don't lose at all, even though I'm trying just as hard as I did at the beginning of the diet. I think the fight's gone out of me. I think I'm done dieting. Hey look, I lost nearly 40 pounds. That's good enough for me.

Maybe it is good enough for Brian. Then again, maybe it isn't. If you, like Brian, seem to be near your goal but find yourself at a standstill, double-check the weight chart and consult with your doctor to make sure there was no error in computing your weight goal. Then ask yourself these questions: Have I set too ambitious a goal? Did I forget to adjust my weight goal as I grew? Am I following the diet guidelines closely enough? Am I physically active enough? If the answers don't give you a clear reason for your inability to lose more weight, then you probably are at the weight that is best for you. In that case, congratulations, you have done a fantastic job in losing all that weight. On the other hand, don't give up too soon. Don't settle for a different weight goal simply because it's an easy way out of further dieting. With that kind of attitude, a marathon runner, after more than twenty-five grueling, pain-racked miles, would give up just a mile short of the finish line.

Carmen, fifteen, lost 77 pounds and was 5 pounds from her goal: It's been hard for me to lose these final five pounds. I know that no one can tell the difference if I lose the five pounds or not. But reaching my goal is so important to me.

Being a winner requires more than learning the do's and don'ts of the diet. Following its guidelines may seem fairly easy when you read them. But putting them into practice out in the real world is another matter. You must be able to deal with temptation. You must be able to recover from mistakes. You must be able to handle your diet in less than ideal situations such as in school, at parties, and on holidays. In other words, you must be able to cope.

Coping on the Diet

13

COPING WITH TEMPTATION

Temptation. There's no escaping it. Watch your favorite TV program and . . . bingo . . . on comes a commercial asking, "Aren't you hungry?" Read your favorite magazines and . . . pop . . . there's a recipe for a gooey dessert. Listen to your favorite radio station and . . . zap . . . the D.J. is talking about a local club's all-you-can-eat spaghetti dinner. On the school grounds, kids are munching on candy bars. At home, your brothers and sisters are attacking chocolate cake. You can't avoid temptation unless you want to hole up on a deserted island and have your family parachute your food to you.

The world is not going to change because you are on a diet. Bakers are still going to make cream-filled pastries and honey-glazed doughnuts. Supermarkets are still going to carry potato chips and cookies. Your thin friends are still going to eat ice cream cones and cheeseburgers. Restaurants are still going to serve cream sauces and rich gravies.

That means you must face temptation square on—and beat it. After a few successes, you soon discover that temptation is not so strong an enemy. You have the power to defeat it. Of course, there's no sense in walking into difficult situations if they can be sidestepped.

Short of chaining up your refrigerator door and padlocking the cupboards, you and your family can help your cause considerably by outlawing fattening junk foods in the house. At the very least, work out an arrangement with your family to keep these foods far from anyone's reach, perhaps in the back part of the kitchen cabinet.

Have you ever heard the old saying, "An idle mind is the devil's playground"? That holds true for dieters. If you have time on your hands, temptation is more likely to bedevil you. So get involved with life—and living. Set your own pace, but fill up your free time so you are too busy even to think about food. Try extracurricular activities at school, start a new hobby, or get a part-time job (no, not at a burger joint). The more active you are, the more enjoyment you get out of life, and the less important food becomes to you. If food loses its importance, temptation loses its strength.

The simplest thing (although not necessarily the easiest) is to shut your mouth, snub your nose, and turn your back on whatever fattening food is tempting you. That sounds good until you are staring at a mouth-watering dessert. When you are in that situation, try this: Ask yourself, "How much happiness can I get from eating this dessert? Each bite is in my mouth for only a few seconds and then it slides down into my stomach. It will make me fatter and undo all the good I've accomplished on the diet. Is that one moment really worth it?"

Some battles with temptation require imagination on your part. So take a few more seconds to create a mental picture in your mind that can help you fight back. Close your eyes, take a deep breath, and imagine exactly how you will feel if you eat the dessert. Think about the awful stuffed feeling you must endure as your stomach bloats and churns from the fattening food. Think about the blubber bulging even more around your belly and hips like an inner tube. Think about the sluggishness and laziness you feel afterward. It's hardly a pretty picture.

COPING WITH TEMPTATION   145

Rick, twelve, lost 12 pounds and was 3 pounds from his goal: When I want a snack that I shouldn't have, I make up something really gross, like that the snack came from the bottom of a smelly garbage can where rats and flies were eating.

Patty, fourteen, lost 14 pounds and was 11 pounds from her goal: When I'm faced with temptation, I imagine that the food will give me zits. I picture my face breaking out all over and grease oozing out of my pores. It's real yucky to think about that, isn't it? But it works for me.

You don't have to conjure up ugly visions that make you want to gag. Use your imagination to create positive, inspiring mental pictures too.

Don, seventeen, lost 24 pounds and was 53 pounds from his goal: I know what I do when I'm tempted. I think about the person I want to be. I have this image of what I want to look like at my goal. I'm at the beach and I have a trim new body. I'm not wearing a shirt and I have this great tan and a girl on each arm. I intend to be that person and I know I never will if I give in to temptation.

When temptation rears its awful head, try to buy some time. Before taking that bite, do something else first for a few minutes.

Randi, fourteen, lost 21 pounds and was 6 pounds from her goal: I really had a craving for a cupcake, so I went to the cupboard and opened a package. But instead of eating it, I set it down on the counter and told myself, "I really want that cupcake, but I'll go do something else first and if in ten minutes I still want it, I'll come back and eat it." I returned ten minutes later and I still wanted that cupcake but not quite as badly, so I held out for another ten minutes. When I returned again, I took the cupcake and threw it in the garbage, and just to make sure I wouldn't fish it out, I dumped ashes from an ashtray over it.

Brad, thirteen, lost 18 pounds and was 10 pounds from his goal: When I want to eat something that's bad for me, I run upstairs to my bedroom and try to get into the outfit that I bought for the day when I reach my goal. I'm getting closer to the day when I can get into it. That gives me encouragement and I lay off the wrong food.

Julie, thirteen, lost 14 pounds and was 11 pounds from her goal: I have a real big sweet tooth and sometimes I get a craving like you wouldn't believe. If I want to get some candy, I go and brush my teeth instead. It helps take away my taste for sweets.

Many young people are aware that temptation can strike at any moment—and they are prepared with their own "emergency kit" or special pep talk.

Marianne, fifteen, lost 18 pounds and was 12 pounds from her goal: I always carry a picture of me that was taken just before I went on the diet. When I'm tempted, I pull it out. One look is all I need. I know if I eat something I shouldn't, I will always look like that picture—or even worse.

Jacqui, thirteen, lost 17 pounds and was 7 pounds from her goal: In my purse is a full-page ad that I tore out of a magazine and folded up. It shows a pretty girl in a cute blouse and tight jeans. I want to look like her. When I have a problem with temptation, I get the ad out and look at it.

Tim, fifteen, lost 35 pounds and was 20 pounds from his goal: Before the diet, I had a habit of snooping around in the refrigerator and I always managed to find something to eat. When I first started to diet, I stood in front of the refrigerator and drooled over the food I couldn't have. Then I wised up after a couple of months. I got out a photograph of me that was taken before I went on the diet and I taped it to the refrigerator door. Now that helps me.

Ron, sixteen, lost 22 pounds and was 21 pounds from his goal: If there is something I want and I know it's not on my diet, I tell myself, "Would my dog eat this?" If the answer is yes, I give it to him. If the answer is no, I throw it away because why should I eat something that even a dog wouldn't eat?

Occasionally, kind-hearted (but sometimes unthinking) people are going to tempt you with food. They might say something like, "Go ahead and take it. One won't hurt you." They are wrong.

If you eat one potato chip, then you might think it's okay to eat one ice cream cone and then eat one plate of spaghetti, and before you know it, you have one big fat problem. Don't give in to the "just one" syndrome. If you eat "just one" bite of apple pie or "just one" bite of a candy bar, you could easily take another bite and another and before you come to your senses, you won't believe you ate the whole thing.

Stephanie, sixteen, lost 22 pounds and was 15 pounds from her goal: Friends who want you to eat something bad for you and say "Go ahead, I won't tell anyone you ate it," are not your friends. They may not tell anyone, but you have to live with it—on your hips. If you think of your diet as a game, you are going to have problems staying away from the wrong kinds of food. Dieting is so serious to me that I won't give in, no matter what other people say or what junk food they tempt me with. I want to be thinner and junk food isn't going to get in my way. I've worked too hard to lose weight and I'm not going to blow it because a friend offers me some brownies.

Sometimes you may need to talk to somebody about how you feel. You may want to share your problems or seek support in moments of weakness. Don't hide your feelings. Talk them out with someone you trust: "I really want to eat fish and chips but I know I can't." "I'm trying to stick to the diet but sometimes it seems so hard." "It's not fair that you can eat anything you want and not gain a pound, and I have to diet."

In my classes, young people talk about food all the time. You might think they are punishing or torturing themselves when they describe meals and desserts. But actually, by talking it out, they vent any frustration and gain strength to fight temptation. It's only natural that you miss certain foods or that you are tempted. Go ahead and recall those days when you made little sculptures with your hot fudge sundae or dug craters in your mashed potatoes and filled them with gravy. If you are struggling with temptation, turn to someone for help—a friend, your parents, a special relative.

Sarah, fourteen, lost 21 pounds and was 20 pounds from her goal: When I am ready to give in to temptation, I'll talk about it to anyone who will listen. I have a girlfriend who is on the diet. When I want to eat something not on the diet, I call her up and say, "Let's chew the fat." That's our signal that I need help. When she's facing temptation, she calls me. We've helped each other stick with the diet.

Don, seventeen, lost 24 pounds and was 53 pounds from his goal: You shouldn't be ashamed about talking to others about the diet. Everybody is dieting anyway, so if I am having trouble with temptation, I talk it out with a friend who can offer me support. I think it helps to diet with a friend.

Temptation often lurks in the homes of latchkey students who return from school to an empty house. Imagine being in the kitchen alone with all that food in the cupboards and refrigerator. It's just you and a piece of apple pie. If you did sneak a piece of pie, nobody would know. But you would know. And the mirror and scale will not let you forget it either.

During the two or three hours before the rest of the family comes home, there are several things you could be doing instead of risking temptation. Get your homework done. Gab on the phone or invite your friend over. Stay occupied.

Diana, fifteen, lost 20 pounds and was 12 pounds from her goal: My job is to clean the house when I come home from school. I do all the other rooms first and I leave the kitchen for last because that's where the temptation is the greatest. Mom comes home from work about the time I start in the kitchen. I have no problem with temptation while I cook or prepare meals with Mom. She gives me the support I need, especially when I have weak moments and I want to give in to temptation.

Another place where temptation beckons you is the fast food restaurant where your friends hang out after school. You may want to be with your friends even though they are chomping on fries and slurping soft drinks. Join them if you want but try not to eat. Or sit down with them and drink an iced tea or a diet soda and gnaw on a piece of fruit that you saved from lunch. If you think you won't be able to resist the temptation to eat something you shouldn't, try to arrange to meet elsewhere, such as at your house or in the park.

Michael, sixteen, lost 18 pounds and was 34 pounds from his goal: I went to McDonald's with my friends and it was a mistake. I ordered just a diet soda and before long I was eating a little of everyone else's french fries. One of my friends said,

"I thought you were on a diet." And I mumbled something like, "Yeah, well I deserve a break today." Before I left, I ate a Big Mac, large order of fries, and an ice cream sundae. I was really a wreck. I gave in and I did it in front of all my friends. That was the pits for me. I know my limitations. I can't go into a fast food place without torturing myself. So I have to stay away from them. Sometimes that means not being with my friends. Sometimes that's a tough choice to make.

Junk foods that you think you can't live without—and are still temptations to you—eventually lose much of their appeal. That's because on a low-salt, low-sugar diet, your taste buds may change and you acquire new tastes. After a few months on the diet, sweets taste too sweet and salty foods taste too salty.

Kevin, twelve, lost 17 pounds and was 7 pounds from his goal: My friend opened up a bag of pretzels at lunch and offered me some. They had always been a favorite snack and I couldn't say no, even though I had been on the diet for two months. I took one bite and I couldn't believe it. It tasted so salty I spit it out. It was hard to imagine how I could have ever liked them.

You soon discover that after a few weeks on the diet, you are making the right choices about what you eat. Temptation becomes less of a problem because your determination to reach your goal increases. As a result, you are able to go into a grocery store and walk right past the cookie and candy aisles without blinking an eye. And if you do stop for a moment in front of the frozen dessert display case, you might say, "That's the food that made me fat," and walk away. You end up with a renewed sense of commitment and power—the power to maintain control of your life and overcome temptations. It's a great feeling!

14
COPING IN SCHOOL

Striving for good grades in school is tough enough without the added responsibility of sticking to a diet. Like others on the diet, you probably face teasing in the classroom and temptation in the lunchroom. How well you handle these challenges can determine your success or failure in reaching your goal. Fortunately, those who maintain the proper attitude, composure, and determination can learn to cope with any diet-related hassles at school.

You've probably been called fatty, chubby, horse, elephant, or whale—you name it. That's the price you pay for being fat. One minor consolation is that every other fat person has been called the same names, so you are not alone. That may not seem like much help to you, but keep in mind that all of the young people in my classes who reached their goals were once teased and called names. They learned to cope and so can you. Your best bet is to find ways to prevent trouble from brewing. Here are some suggestions:

Keep a low profile about your diet. Sure, it's okay to confide in a friend if you want, but don't advertise to the whole school that you are on a diet. Otherwise you risk the chance of being teased even more about dieting than about being overweight.

Be nice to others. Compliment them on their appearance, their good grades, or some achievement. Who's going to tease you if you make them feel good?

Participate in various school functions. Join groups and organizations. They are perfect opportunities for others to get to know you better and to accept you as a person.

> *Terri, sixteen, lost 24 pounds and was 29 pounds from her goal:* I seldom get teased and I think I know why. I've always had a cheerful personality and I'm into a lot of after-school activities. I've made a lot of friends that way. Friends won't deliberately hurt me or say mean things to me.

Have a sense of humor. People like to hang around others who make them smile. Also, a sense of humor takes the steam out of any teasing. If you can laugh it off, people are less likely to tease you.

> *Don, seventeen, lost 24 pounds and was 53 pounds from his goal:* If you don't have a sense of humor, you could end up in deep trouble. I crack fat jokes sometimes and poke fun at myself because that way the others laugh with me, not at me. Basically, I've beaten them to the punch so they don't bother teasing me.

Look as good as you can. Always wear clean, neat clothes, comb your hair, and stand up straight. When you show others you care about yourself, you are less likely to become the target of teasers.

> *Joshua, fifteen, lost 18 pounds and was 24 pounds from his goal:* If you look like a slob, you get treated like a slob. People

tease slobs. That's why I'm always well groomed and neatly dressed. I'm no Joe Cool and I don't pretend to be, but looking nice and neat is very important to me. I look as good as possible and work extra hard at it because appearance means a lot to people.

Sometimes you can't prevent the teasing because you can't hide the fact that you are fat, even though you are doing everything possible to lose weight. Patience and a positive attitude are important traits to develop to keep you from falling off the diet.

Heidi, thirteen, lost 24 pounds and was 11 pounds from her goal: Kids would tease me and sing "Roll, roll, roll your fat." It hurt but I knew that if I could trim down, I wouldn't hear teasing anymore. Every time I was teased I put that much more effort into the diet, and now I'm almost there.

Your determination to succeed can't be based on other people's opinions. They didn't make you fat and they didn't make you go on this diet. You started the diet because you, and only you, want to better yourself. I know it's easier said than done, but don't worry about what people think of your dieting. Stick with it and be what you want to be. Don't let others dictate your life.

Sarah, fourteen, lost 31 pounds and reached her goal: I was always called names at school, like every day of my life it seemed. I didn't cope very well and it was so awful that I didn't want to go to school. When I started the diet, I kept thinking the name-calling would stop, but it didn't. I guess they were used to seeing me fat and they knew the teasing would get me upset. But I made up my mind that my day was coming. After I lost 15 pounds, I was still teased. That really bothered me but I knew I could reach my goal and I wasn't going to let some cruel remarks stop me. Finally, when I reached my goal, I wore a pair of designer jeans with a beautiful sweater tucked in. I wore my hair down and restyled it, used eye makeup, and made my splash. The comments and compliments from the former teasers seemed very hollow to me. I discovered that these people acted like a bunch of space cadets and airheads and I didn't really care whether they liked the way I looked or not. My real friends—the ones who stuck by me and encouraged me through thick and thin—raved about how great I looked. I only wish I hadn't let the teasing get to me for so long during the diet.

Some young people try to blunt the teaser's barbs by saying, "Yes, I know I'm fat. And I'm trying to do something about it." You just won't be able to shut some people up. The more you try to explain, the more they will put you down. Sometimes it's best not to say anything at all and to walk away from the situation.

Sometimes the teasing gets so hot you are ready to boil over. Don't pick a fight with the teaser because you can't win. You either get beaten up, in which case you suffer further teasing and humiliation, or you beat up the other person and gain a reputation as a bully. Furthermore, you could end up in serious trouble with the school authorities.

Bob, fifteen, lost 15 pounds and was 25 pounds from his goal: I've been called names like "fatso" and "blubbo" and that gets me real mad. The others know that so they keep it up. But I no longer take it like I used to. Last month I just exploded and duked it out with one of the creeps. I gave him a black eye and I didn't get hurt. But we were both suspended from school for a week.

Don't scheme for ways to get even with the teaser. One common ploy is to dwell on some imperfection of the teaser. You know what I mean. First you mention to others that Suzy has a big nose and before long Suzy is called Pinocchio. She's humiliated and you feel smug. Or do you? Eventually you end up feeling bad, because you realize you are no better than the teaser. You have lowered yourself to the teaser's level. That's not too smart, considering the fact that with this diet you are aiming to reach new heights in personal achievement and self-improvement.

If you have a bad day at school because you are teased, the first urge is to rush home and raid the refrigerator because that's what you used to do. Think before you go off the deep end and dive into a mound of ice cream to soothe your pain. Okay, so somebody hurt your feelings by telling you he can't see how you lost eighteen pounds because you don't look it. Instead of having a binge, ask yourself: Is it really worth it? Does that person's opinion mean so much to you that you're willing to fall off the diet?

In the days before you started the diet, you used to believe that food made you feel secure and good. Now, though, you know that eating the wrong foods in the wrong way has the opposite effect. Eating out of anger or frustration can make you feel guilty and depressed, not to mention fatter.

Charlie was a twelve-year-old whom the other students called Orca the Whale because he was about fifty pounds overweight. Naturally, he hated the name and let everyone know it, which made the students call him Orca that much more. Whenever he was upset, he'd run home and devour a big bowl of ice cream or a huge hunk of cake. The more he ate, the fatter he got. The fatter he got, the more he was teased. The more he was teased, the more he ate. He was trapped in a vicious cycle.

You can avoid falling into the same trap. If you are hurt and angry from the teasing at school, hustle off to your room at home and scream, punch your pillow, pound your fists into the mattress. Walk or jog around the block. Do anything to work out your frustration. Keeping it all bottled up can lead to overeating.

Melissa, thirteen, lost 41 pounds and reached her goal: I'd get teased at school and I'd take it without saying a word. I'd wait until I'd get home and then I let it all out. I'd scream and rant and rave and really get worked up. Fortunately, I have a great mom and she understood and let me get out all my bad feelings. Then we'd talk about it and I'd feel so much better. She kept saying, "Wait until you reach your goal and everything will be better." She was right.

Although good friends give you needed encouragement and support throughout the diet, certain other friends—whether they mean to or not—may actually try to push you off the diet. Some may think you are suffering on the diet and that you deserve a little treat, so they may urge you to go ahead and eat that piece of cake or have that cookie.

Vance, fourteen, lost 34 pounds and reached her goal: Don't give in to your friends. Sometimes they want to be nice guys so they try to share fattening food with you. When they offer things like that to me, I tell them if they care about me they shouldn't give me food. Then I try to change the subject and ask them to go for a bike ride or go for a walk or listen to the stereo. Sometimes it's harder to keep your friends' minds off food than it is to stop thinking about it yourself.

What do you do with a fat friend who tries to ruin your attempt to diet? Let's say your friend Linda tries to tempt you with a fattening dessert or claims you don't need to diet. Your friend could be doing this out of jealousy because she doesn't have the determination or drive to attempt to improve herself. Linda could also be sabotaging your diet out of fear, afraid of being left behind while you go on to a slim, new life. She won't have anyone with whom to share her fudge or split a pizza. Worse yet, she will have to fend off the teasers alone. She'd much rather have you as company so both of you can be fat and miserable together. Remember, misery loves company.

To combat this, talk over your feelings with Linda. Tell

her that you would be happy to share the diet with her and that by slimming down together you can offer each other support. Even if she doesn't want to diet, show her that you care and tell her that you won't think any less of her just because she can't or won't lose weight. Assure her that you will still be friends. But make her understand that the days of pigging out together are over. And ask her to show support by not trying to ruin your diet.

Unfortunately, there may even be thin students who tease you, not only for what they consider the fun of it but also because they want to see you fail. They may stick a candy bar under your nose or eat a piece of cake in front of you. These kids hate to see anyone be successful because they don't have what it takes to succeed. They don't have enough determination or ambition to improve whatever it is about themselves that needs changing. So instead of attempting to reach your lofty level, they prefer to try to drag you down to theirs.

It's like teasing the class brain—the one who *never* gives the wrong answer. Some students want to knock the class brain down a notch or two, wishing that just once he or she would get an "F" on an exam.

Coping with temptation during lunch at school can seem difficult when you begin the diet. It's not easy to watch other students in the cafeteria eating fattening meals or junk food. It's not easy until you realize that your lunch of raw vegetables, fruit, and a thick pita bread sandwich is helping you slim down.

When the teasers see that your brown bag no longer bulges from hoagies, cupcakes, and potato chips, you could be the target of diet jokes. So how do you cope in the cafeteria? You can move to another table, eat with students who are also dieting, or have lunch with supportive friends. To anyone who has commented negatively about your diet, show them exactly what you are eating. You could even bring extra vegetables and fruit for others to sample. You may soon notice that some of those same students who were teasing you and joking about the diet are now bringing their own pita bread sandwiches and slices of fruit and vegetables. But some people never change, so learn to ignore them.

> *Sandra, twelve, lost 23 pounds and was 25 pounds from her goal:* One girl kept teasing me at lunch. One day I was eating my pita bread sandwich and she was sticking an ice cream bar under my nose, saying, "Don't you wish you could have this?" She kept it up until I had enough. I grabbed the ice cream bar out of her hand and threw it in the garbage. I never had any more trouble from her after that.

Although this worked for Sandra, I don't believe in throwing anyone else's food away. To help you cope with being tempted by all the fattening food around you, think of your lunch period as a time for things other than just eating. Use some of those minutes as a break from the classroom routine. Socialize with friends, relax, or read a book. You don't necessarily have to spend your whole lunch period in the cafeteria eating. In fact, if your school rules allow it, try eating your lunch picnic style outside under a tree or on a bench.

If you can manage coping with your lunch period, you can handle temptation brought on by other school events such as bake sales, candy sales, carnivals, and football games. As I've said before, it's important for you to enjoy the activity for what it is, not for the food involved. Obviously, don't go out of your way to be tempted. It should go without saying that if you volunteer to work in a booth at the school carnival, choose a booth that has nothing to do with food, such as the ring toss. You are courting possible dieting disaster if you work the cake walk or the soft drink concession.

If you must sell candy to raise money for the school

band, stay cool. View each candy bar as a piece of merchandise, nothing more, and you shouldn't have any problem. There may be times when you feel compelled to buy candy because the money is going to a good cause. Just make sure that candy is not going to a bad cause—your stomach. There's nothing wrong with buying candy if you plan to give it away immediately.

Jason, fourteen, lost 22 pounds and was 13 pounds from his goal: As a prize for selling so many magazines during our fundraiser at school, I was given all sorts of candy. I really wanted to eat it, but then I thought there was no way. It wasn't easy for me, though, especially when some of my friends were eating their prizes. Between classes I took the candy and passed it out to some of the girls I like.

Remember, try your best to prevent teasing and temptations from testing your determination in school. Keep a low profile about your diet, have a sense of humor, be nice to others, and look as good as you can. If you are teased, be cool and stick to the diet. The sooner you reach your goal, the sooner the teasing should stop.

15

COPING ON HOLIDAYS AND AT SPECIAL EVENTS

No matter what the holiday, it seems as though you are caught in a twenty-four-hour blitz of table-bending dinner spreads, tantalizing snacks, and mouth-watering, home-baked goodies. Unfortunately, too many people view holidays as opportunities to stuff themselves silly with food.

However, since no one is going to change the way the majority of the country treats holidays, I think it's in your best interest to let up on your diet on certain special occasions. It's asking too much of you to eat only what's on the diet while the rest of the family is savoring a delicious holiday feast. During times like these you could feel pretty low eating foods different from what everyone else is enjoying because you are fat and on a diet. And if you did eat what they ate, then you'd feel miserable because you fell off the diet. So what do you do?

Declare the holiday an Ease-up Day. That's a time when you make some adjustments to the diet so you can enjoy the holiday meal with the rest of the family. It's just for one festive occasion, and these occur only a few times during the year, on such days as Thanksgiving, Christmas, or Passover. You can also include no more than one or two other special events such as your bar mitzvah, your graduation celebration, or a wedding.

An Ease-up Day is not a shut-your-mind-open-your-mouth kind of day in which you gobble everything in sight like a berserk Pac-Man. You are still very much on the diet and must practice all the good eating habits you have learned. However, on an Ease-up Day you can sample other foods that you normally wouldn't eat while on the diet.

For example, if you make Thanksgiving an Ease-up Day, you can eat what everyone else at the table eats: turkey, cranberry sauce, vegetables with a cheese sauce, a roll, mashed potatoes and gravy, stuffing, salad, and a piece of pumpkin pie.

You're probably drooling already just picturing the meal in your mind, right? But you still must follow several guidelines:

Eat the low-calorie food first. For example, eat your salad first, and then the turkey, so that you are filling up on food that has helped you slim down. Then try some of the other foods. Leave the fattening foods for last so that if you are almost full by the time you are ready to eat them, you tend to eat less of them.

Eat in moderation. Take one roll, not two. Try a small helping of mashed potatoes, not a whole plateful. Eat one thin piece of pie, not a giant wedge. And no second helpings are allowed. On an Ease-up Day, you can enjoy a taste of the same foods that everyone else is eating. Don't use the holiday as an excuse to binge.

Do not starve yourself the day before or the day after the holiday. Stick with your diet up until the moment of your holiday dinner and then return to the diet after the meal. Don't do anything different to prepare for the Ease-up Day.

Do not eat junk food or candy. The basic reason for Ease-up Days is to allow you to enjoy with your family food specially prepared for a specific occasion. It does not give you the license to eat common, everyday junk food and candy.

Do as much physical activity as you can during the holiday. Try to burn up extra calories through such activities as a brisk after-dinner walk since you will be consuming more calories than usual.

Do not feel guilty. You have not fallen off the diet. You have not cheated. Instead, you have made an adjustment in your food choices for one particular holiday dinner. It's okay. You should feel more self-confident because you can prove to yourself that you are in control. Think back to the last big holiday dinner before you started the diet. You probably ate half a pie that day. This holiday, you are content to taste just a sliver of pie.

Bear in mind that Ease-up Days don't come free. You do pay a price. And only you can decide if it's worth it. The cost will show up when you step on the scale at the end of the week. It's likely that you will not have lost any weight and in fact may have gained a pound. Don't fret about it. Accept it and go on with your diet. Again, don't feel guilty about it. A chronic case of the guilts can trigger an eating binge.

Also, your body may protest on the day after an Ease-up Day. All the rich, high-calorie food you ate could make you feel somewhat lousy physically and give you a stomachache or headache.

Stephen, fifteen, lost 43 pounds and was 24 pounds from his goal. A year ago I started pigging out at Thanksgiving and I didn't quit until after New Year's Day. I mean, I ate every kind of Christmas cookie, pie, cake, and nut bread you can name. I helped my mom make ten dozen giant-size Toll

House cookies to give as gifts to our neighbors and within a week I ate most of them. My mom yelled at me for hours about how fat I was and that I had no self-control. I felt the worst ever in my whole life. I went on the diet a few weeks later. This past Christmas season I didn't gain an ounce because all that stuff wasn't important to me like it once was. I ate some things not on the diet during the Ease-up Day but they were only a nibble compared to a binge.

As best you can, turn your attention away from food during the Thanksgiving to New Year holiday season. Try to find ways other than cooking to celebrate these special days. Instead of being tantalized by all the wonderful aromas in the kitchen, go outside and collect different colored leaves, pine cones, and nuts and make a centerpiece for the dinner table, or make some seasonal decorations. Atmosphere, as much as food, can make the holiday seem much brighter for everyone.

If you do make food such as cookies for holiday gifts, then package them right away. Seal the jars or boxes, wrap them up, and get them to your friends and neighbors. But instead of giving food treats, why not make Christmas decorations or other knickknacks? Find things that keep you busy throughout Christmas vacation. Help decorate a nursing home or go caroling.

Margie, thirteen, lost 30 pounds and reached her goal: Last Christmas was a real downfall for me. I don't understand why everyone makes so much food for just one day. I gained eight pounds during Christmas vacation because it was food, food, food. This Christmas is different. I'm staying very busy making my own Christmas cards, knitting stockings to hang by the fireplace, and I'm part of a group that is making holiday favors to put on trays for patients in the hospital. I'm having fun and I feel good about myself. Also, I'm giving others a happy holiday that has nothing to do with food.

Sarah, fourteen, lost 41 pounds and reached her goal: I had a real tame Christmas while on the diet. I still baked things but instead of eating them I gave them away as part of a food basket program for the poor. When I thought about the people here in town who are hungry, somehow my problem of overeating seemed pretty dumb.

Gene, thirteen, lost 22 pounds and was 9 pounds from his goal: My cousins and I all go to the same school so we decided to get together and do a play for the whole family for Thanksgiving. We wrote it and made costumes and some props and then on Thanksgiving we gave the play. It was a funny one about the history of our family. All the relatives loved it. It was the best Thanksgiving because we all had such a good time. For once, dinner wasn't the main event—at least not to me.

Other holidays can be celebrated without easing up on the diet. Although Halloween probably ranks right near the top as a favorite holiday, it doesn't qualify as an Ease-up Day. Nevertheless, you can still have plenty of fun on Halloween without toppling off the diet.

You want to trick or treat? Go right ahead and fill your bag with candy bars, suckers, gum, and caramels. Just make sure you give it all away. The fun should come from dressing up in costume, not from eating the goodies. Distributing your candy to a nearby nursing home or a hospital or giving it to the lonely widow down the street will make you feel good about yourself. Just get the candy out of the house as soon as possible.

If candy in the house before and after Halloween presents a temptation for you, ask your mother if you can pick out the candy that is to be given away to the trick or treaters. Then choose the candy that you can't stand. Maybe it's licorice or peppermint. Better yet, buy nonfood treats. You can pass out such things as stickers, pencils, erasers, or nickels. You'll discover that you can have fun on Halloween without thinking about candy at all.

> *Rick, twelve, lost 12 pounds and was 3 pounds from his goal:* I didn't go out for Halloween this year because I didn't want to be tempted. Instead, some buddies and I set up a haunted house in my garage and charged the neighborhood kids a dime. We had a graveyard scene outside and spooky sounds that we taped and played over the stereo. Inside the haunted house we had kids dressed up in all sorts of weird costumes to scare everyone. In one dark room we made the kids stick their hands in bowls of things like peeled grapes and cold, greasy macaroni and we told them they were touching eyeballs and snakes. I had so much fun I never thought about candy or sweets.

The summer holidays such as Memorial Day, the Fourth of July, and Labor Day are usually geared to picnics and cookouts. That's easy to cope with because you can bring your own cooler filled with all the things you need to eat. Instead of chips and dip, you can share your chilled vegetables and a low-calorie dip. There's nothing wrong with cooking a hamburger patty, chicken franks, or chicken breast on a barbecue grill. If one of the summer holidays is a big event in your family, then make it an Ease-up Day. Enjoy sampling the spread of food, but again, make sure you eat in moderation and eat the least fattening things first. These are the days for physical activities such as swimming, softball, and volleyball. Don't sit next to the food. Get out and play hard.

16

COPING AT PARTIES

You have just been invited to a party Saturday night and you readily accept. But your excitement quickly dwindles because you are on a diet. "Looks like it won't be much fun after all if I stick to my diet," you tell yourself. "And if I go off my diet, then I'll feel miserable."

Hold on a minute. With that kind of thinking, you are better off living in solitary confinement. Don't punish yourself. There's no reason in the world why you can't have a great time. So what if you are on a diet? It shouldn't make any difference—no more than if you are a lefthander or a Capricorn or a brunette.

Stop and think what parties are: a gathering of friends for fun. People don't attend parties just for the food. When you ask your friends to recall the great times they've had at parties, it's highly unlikely that their recollections include any mention of food, unless it comes as an afterthought.

Unfortunately, some dieters miss the whole point of what a party is supposed to be. Their problem is that they equate fun with food. They act as though a party has no meaning unless their mouths and stomachs are full; as if they can't even carry on an intelligent or witty conversation without their hands in the chips and dip; as if dancing is merely a series of three-minute breaks from the snacks. You are at the party to have a good time. So have a good time. Focus your attention on the other kids, the music, and the fun.

One way to make it easier on yourself is to eat before you go to a party. Don't go on an empty stomach. If you are offered food that could wreck your diet, politely refuse. Some young people in my classes admit that they make up excuses to the host such as "I'm allergic to chocolate," or "I'm a diabetic so I can't eat cake." Forget the phony stories and simply say, "No, thank you." No explanation is needed. If the host persists, then you might want to say, "Thanks very much but there are only certain things I can eat, and this is not one of them." It often helps if you ask for something that your diet permits, such as iced tea or unbuttered popcorn. That makes the other person feel that he or she is being a good host. Don't make a big deal about refusing food. No one is going to think anything less of you.

If you want to keep your diet a secret, then go ahead and accept the food. (Read carefully—I said *accept*, not eat.) Take the food and then set it somewhere and forget about it. No one is going to pay attention to who is eating and who isn't.

> *Eva, fifteen, lost 22 pounds and was 6 pounds from her goal:* When I'm given a slice of pizza or cake at a party, I take it and then walk over to a boy I want to meet and offer it to him. Then I introduce myself. If someone asks me where my food is, I say that I ate already.

> *Sonia, sixteen, lost 38 pounds and reached her goal:* When I go to a party, I mix and mingle with everyone there. I get the boys to talk about themselves and then they never shut up. I don't pay attention to the food or what other people are eating.

Jason, fourteen, lost 22 pounds and was 13 pounds from his goal: At parties, I don't go near the food. When someone asks if I want something to eat, I say, "Maybe later." If they insist, I take the food and then dump it because I don't want any hassles. No one has caught on to me yet.

Being on a diet is no reason for you not to throw a party, whether you are celebrating your birthday or just looking for a good time. Plan the party around some activity such as bowling, swimming, skating, miniature golf, or a movie. Or hold a bash with a theme such as a Fifties party or a punk rock party. Keep it lively and fun. When people are bored, they tend to drift toward the food table and snack on the goodies just for something to do.

You can serve a wide range of food without making it the highlight of the party. Introduce them to healthy food such as fruit juices, popcorn, pita bread pizza, raw vegetables with dip and a hollowed-out watermelon loaded with slices of fresh fruit that can be speared with toothpicks. People are always looking for new experiences at parties.

Girls in my classes say that of all the parties they attend, slumber parties are the most challenging. But they don't have to be a night-long struggle against temptation— if you are prepared. For instance, when you are invited over for dinner, ask if you can bring over the basic food you need to eat and prepare it there. Another choice is to have dinner at home first and then go to the slumber party. There is nothing wrong with bringing your own bag of goodies to snack on (as long as you have enough to share with others). For the party, contribute a six-pack of diet soda, or a basket of fresh fruit or popcorn.

Elyse, thirteen, lost 18 pounds and was 10 pounds from her goal: When I go to a slumber party, I tell the party-giver I'm on a diet. It seems she goes out of her way to help me. She makes sure she has the right food for me to eat. We're usually having such a good time talking about boys that I don't get upset or tempted when the girls are eating barbecue sandwiches.

The younger you are, the harder it might seem to handle birthday parties while on the diet. Actually, they aren't as difficult as you may think. Remember, you attend parties to have fun, not to eat. Enjoy the games and prizes and the opening of presents. What do you do when it's time for the cake and ice cream? In certain cases you may feel most comfortable simply accepting the cake and ice cream. Just don't eat it.

If you don't mind that others know you are bettering yourself by dieting, try another approach. Seek the help of the parent who is throwing the birthday party and explain that you are on a diet. Most parents are very understanding.

Laura, eleven, lost 24 pounds and reached her goal: I don't know where I got the nerve, but the day before the party I called my friend's mother and told her I was on a special diet and that I couldn't have cake and ice cream, soda, or candy. They were going to grill hamburgers and have potato chips, so I asked if they could make me a small one. Marsha's mother said not to worry. They were so nice to me at the party. The other kids were given little baskets of candy bars and I got a little basket of grapes and strawberries. They gave me a small hamburger without the bun and some raw vegetables and diet soda. The other kids had hamburgers, chips, and soda. I ate my fruit for dessert and the kids had cake and ice cream. I had a good time. Everyone was so understanding. I really enjoyed the birthday party because of the games and prizes and fun. Before, when I went to parties, I'd sit at a table and do nothing but eat and eat.

If you are celebrating your own birthday with a party, you don't have to deprive yourself of cake and ice cream. Consider the day an Ease-up Day. Go ahead and eat a thin slice of cake and one scoop of ice cream if you must. If your party includes lunch or dinner, you can eat foods that are not necessarily on the diet, such as tacos or chili. But skip the junk food and eat in moderation.

No matter what your age or what kind of party you attend, being on a diet should have no bearing on the amount of fun you have.

Katey, fourteen, lost 32 pounds and reached her goal: I wasn't invited to any parties when I was fat, so I didn't have to cope with that. But now that I've lost weight, I'm invited to parties. Coping is very easy for me. I have so much to catch up on that I'm not interested in food. I'm interested in enjoying myself.

17
COPING IN RESTAURANTS

There is no reason in the world why you can't enjoy eating out at a nice restaurant while you are on the diet. That doesn't mean you can eat anything you want or as much as you want. You are still responsible for sticking very close to the diet. The guidelines that you have learned must be followed.

First, let's clarify one point. This chapter does not deal with fast food joints. I'm talking about restaurants that have place settings and waiters or waitresses who give you menus, take your order, and deliver the food to your table. Restaurants like this have the widest variety of healthy food.

Try to find out ahead of time what the restaurant serves so that you won't have a problem once you get there. If it's a restaurant that you have never been to before, call first. Otherwise read the menu if it's posted outside, or ask to see a menu before you are seated, so you are assured there is enough of the kind of food you are allowed.

It helps to go to the restaurant in the right frame of mind. You are there to enjoy the atmosphere, the company, and a break from the routine of eating at home. Food should not dominate your mind.

For many young people, the hardest part of eating in a restaurant is ordering. They are afraid to ask that the food be served in a certain way. Let's get one thing straight: You have the right—no, the responsibility—to request that your meal be prepared to your satisfaction. Don't be bullied by the waiter. It is his job to please you. After all, you (or your parents) are paying for the meal.

Don't be afraid to ask questions about how certain foods are prepared. Does the ground sirloin come with a mushroom sauce? Is the fish fried? Is the veal sautéed in butter? The more knowledgeable you are about the restaurant's food, the better able you are to eat a meal that is right for you. Tell the waiter exactly how you want your meal prepared. Tell him to broil the fish instead of frying it, forget the cheese sauce on the broccoli, and serve the baked potato without butter and sour cream. Tell him the size of the portions you want, too. If any part of your meal is not served the way you asked, send it back.

Lenny, thirteen, lost 18 pounds and was 10 pounds from his goal: At first I was very shy about asking for changes. But at this one small neighborhood restaurant that we go to regularly, my parents urged me to speak up. So I did. I had a super waiter. He excused himself for a second and returned with the cook. After I talked with him, he said to leave everything to him. Out came a terrific meal that tasted great and fit perfectly with the diet. I felt like a million bucks. Now we go there twice a month and the waiter always checks my progress on the diet.

Jeff, fifteen, lost 15 pounds and was 10 pounds from his goal: My parents are great ones for going out to eat at least once a week. It's a family tradition. When I started on the diet, I thought about just staying home because I thought it would be a real drag if I went to a restaurant and wasn't able to order all the things I used to eat. I've always enjoyed restaurants—maybe that's one of the reasons why I have a weight problem—and I didn't want to stay home. So I decided to go out to eat with my parents when the diet began. It wasn't hard at all. I asked the waitress for three ounces of broiled steak, green beans without butter, a plain baked potato, and a tossed salad with low-calorie dressing. She raised her eyebrows but did what I asked. I was very polite and I didn't demand anything from her or the cook. I enjoyed the night out and I have done it several times since.

Debbie, fourteen, lost 31 pounds and was 16 pounds from her goal: I didn't think that I could go out to a restaurant and trust myself. But I found out I can. To help me, I don't look at a menu because it would be too tempting. I just order basic things like broiled chicken and fresh vegetables, and go to the salad bar. I'm surprised to see how restaurants treat young people. The waiters seem to want to please you as much as they can. I'm always courteous because that's how I want people to treat me. I've never experienced a hard time. I also don't go with the idea that I'm being punished since I can't have everything on the menu. I go because it's fun to eat out.

When possible, order à la carte. In other words, order each food item separately rather than selecting a combination plate that includes the entrée and side dishes. By choosing your food items separately, you maintain greater control over how you want your meal to be prepared. (However, à la carte ordering is usually more expensive than selecting a combination plate.)

Take full advantage of salad bars, but don't automatically eat everything that is offered. You know what's good for you and what isn't. Stay away from the creamy dressings, croutons, and bacon bits. When your meal is served, look at the portions. You can tell just by sight how much meat, chicken, or fish you can have. If you are given a six-ounce steak, cut it in half and put half in a doggie bag for lunch or dinner the next day.

Some kids complain that watching others eat food cooked in rich sauces and gravies is pure torture. Torture is in the eye of the beholder. It's agony only if you let it be agony. Enjoy the surroundings, the company, and the conversation. (Besides, you don't have to do the dishes!)

Jillian, twelve, lost 8 pounds and was 25 pounds from her goal: Going to restaurants is hard for me because I want to eat all the foods that I used to eat before going on this diet. A few weeks ago, I went to a restaurant with my parents and I was mad because they could eat anything they wanted and I couldn't. I wanted them to take me home.

People like Jillian who have the wrong attitude face a tough struggle because they view restaurants as a difficult challenge rather than a pleasant experience. If you are going to feel miserable at restaurants, then don't go to them.

Occasionally you might be tempted at a restaurant. Secretly observe (don't stare at) someone in the restaurant who is slender and fits your image of what you want to look like when you reach your goal. Remind yourself that you will look like that some day soon if you stick to your diet. Another way to help you curb temptation is to watch someone nearby who is overweight. Study the way he looks, the way he eats, and what he eats. Do you want to be like him?

For some dieters, dessert time is painful. Everyone is eating some fluffy, sugary pastry or triple-layer cake or mountainous meringue pie. Stick to fresh fruit. Eventually you will get your "just desserts" in the form of a trim body.

Joel, fifteen, lost 23 pounds and was 22 pounds from his goal: Early in my diet, I went out with my parents and their friends to an expensive restaurant. I coped fine until they rolled out the dessert cart right in front of me. I was feeling pretty low as everyone else picked delicious-looking desserts. I really felt left out. I asked the waiter if there were any low-cal desserts and he came back with a beautiful bowl of fresh melon. That perked me up, especially when everyone else at the table wished they had asked for that instead.

18
COPING ON VACATIONS AND AT SUMMER CAMP

Vacations or camp can really do a number on your diet—if you are not prepared. But with a little planning ahead, you can have a fun-filled time without falling off your diet.

Is your family going to drive to the Grand Canyon? To the Badlands? To the Smokies? You can handle such a trip easily while on the diet. If you are going to spend any length of time on the road, take a cooler filled with fruit, vegetables, cheese, pita bread, and iced tea or fruit juices. Eat them on picnics along the way or at your campsite or in your motel room at night. Throughout the trip, stop off at roadside produce stands to buy fresh fruits and vegetables. As you travel to other parts of the country, grab the opportunity to try new tastes—the food and produce that have made the local area or state famous. For example, the state of Washington is famous for its apples, Georgia for its peaches, Wisconsin for its cheese, California for its grapes, and Florida for its oranges.

Part of your vacation fun can come from getting your own food. For instance, if you are an outdoors person, stop off at a calm, tree-lined lake and fish for your dinner. Stroll through pick-your-own groves and pluck fresh fruit directly from the tree. On camping trips, take walks into the woods and collect berries.

Joel, fifteen, lost 23 pounds and was 22 pounds from his goal: We went camping for two weeks in the Smokies. Man, it was fantastic. We hiked every day and that's something I couldn't have handled last year because I was just too fat. What a difference a year makes when you are losing weight. We caught smallmouth bass and brook trout and ate them. We also picked strawberries and, boy, were they good. I had a super time, and best of all, I lost five more pounds.

Sometimes you and your family, because of time and economy, may decide to eat at a fast food restaurant. If at all possible, try to work out an agreement with the rest of the family to at least pick a place where you won't be forced to go off your diet completely. For example, choose a place that offers a salad bar or one that serves tacos. Eaten in moderation (that is, no more than two at a meal), tacos provide a nutritious substitute for a greasy hamburger or fried chicken.

Don't be afraid to speak up about your choice for a fast food place.

Peter, fourteen, lost 32 pounds and was 14 pounds from his goal: I don't get into many difficult situations when we are on vacation because I am very vocal about my diet. If my family wants to go to a pizza place, I say, "No way!" I can't handle that. I've been on the diet for three months and I'm not going to be tempted to go off it because they want pizza. There's nothing for me to eat in a pizza place. It may not seem fair to my family but that's the way it is. We go to some other restaurant.

William, twelve, lost 17 pounds and was 7 pounds from his goal: If I walk into McDonald's there's no way I can stay on my diet. But my family loves McDonald's and that's where we stopped on our way to visit our relatives in North Carolina. We compromised. We went through the drive-in window and they ordered what they wanted and I got a plain hamburger and a diet soda. It wasn't so bad watching my family eat french fries and Quarter Pounders in the car. But if we were in McDonald's, then I wouldn't be able to resist going up to the counter and ordering a bunch of stuff.

If you are caught in a situation where you must either go into a fast food joint or not eat, then make the best of it. Go ahead and eat. But use caution and common sense. For example, order a hamburger with lettuce and tomato. Or get a chicken sandwich and peel off the breading. Or eat a couple of hot dogs without the buns.

If you are staying at a motel and plan on going to a nice restaurant, call ahead first to find out what is on the menu. Then follow the suggestions I mentioned on restaurant eating in chapter 17.

Will you be flying instead of driving? No sweat. You can eat well on an airplane and still stay true blue to the diet. A week or so before your flight, call the airline (or ask your travel agent to phone for you) and request a special low-calorie meal such as a chef's salad or a fruit plate. Almost all airlines are happy to comply and don't charge you anything extra. When you board the plane, remind the flight attendant that you ordered a special meal so you are assured of receiving it. Airlines serve a variety of low-calorie beverages to go with your meal.

Amusement parks can be a strong test of your determination to stick with the diet. But there are a few preventive measures you can take. First, don't go to the park hungry. Make sure you have eaten a good breakfast. Second, bring along a sack lunch or a piece or two of fruit and keep it in your purse or backpack for whenever you get the urge to snack. Third, drink a lot of water throughout the day so your stomach will feel full between meals.

You want to eat something from the concession stand?

Then buy an all-natural frozen juice bar or some unbuttered popcorn. But the most important thing to remember is to enjoy the moment and forget about food. Besides, who can think about food after riding the Cliffhanger or the triple loop Mindbender or the Screaming Eagle?

Summer camp can be an absolute ball or it can be sheer torture. It all depends on picking the right one for you and your diet. Long before you sign up for camp, write to the camp director, explain your situation, and enclose a copy of the diet. Ask if the camp cook can prepare meals that follow the guidelines of the diet or if you can have the opportunity to choose the proper foods offered by a cafeteria-style mess hall. If the camp cannot guarantee you the availability of the right foods, then look for another place to spend part of the summer.

Thomas, thirteen, lost 44 pounds and reached his goal: Last year I hated camp. I had just started the diet and they didn't have any food that was good for me. They lined us up in the mess hall like the army and gave us slop that actually stuck to the spoons and ladles. I didn't eat any of it for the first few days but then I was so starved I ate everything in sight. I got so depressed. I gained ten pounds. This summer I went to a camp in the mountains for eight weeks. I had checked this one out before I went to make sure I wouldn't gain weight because I was almost at my goal by then. I stuck to my diet because I could make my own food choices. They had a variety of dry cereal to choose from each morning and every lunch and dinner had a salad bar. Sure, I went to the canteen every night with the guys, but I honestly wasn't tempted. I just enjoyed being there. I felt good about myself and I joined in different sports. When I got home, I hadn't gained a pound.

Paul, thirteen, lost 23 pounds and was 19 pounds from his goal: Before I went to camp, I wrote and told them how much weight I had lost this past winter. I said I could only go to their camp if they promised to help me by having the proper foods. I was surprised when the camp director called me instead of writing a letter. He asked all about the diet and how I thought the camp could improve in serving the best food possible. Let me tell you, I felt very important. When I went to camp, they had a salad bar and lots of fresh fruits and vegetables and meals specially prepared for people on diets. It made camp so much more fun for me.

Weight reduction camps or "fat farms" are gaining in popularity because their whole program, from the activities to the food, is geared toward the fat young person. Many such campers have lost an impressive amount of weight by the end of their stay. The only problem is that they tend to put it right back on once they are home.

It's easy to lose weight because in many of these camps it's not the real world. There is no Dunkin' Donuts, no Wendy's, no Kentucky Fried Chicken within walking distance. There are no vending machines chock-full of tempting candy bars, corn chips, and soda. There are no little brothers to pester you or parents to nag you. All responsibility is lifted from you. The camp decides your menus and the camp prepares your food. You have little to say about when you eat, what you eat, and how much you exercise.

But it works, you say. That may be true. However, what have you *learned*? Do you know how to continue losing weight at home? Do you know how to maintain your new weight? Do you know the basics of good nutrition? Do you know how to cope with common temptations and hassles? Do you know how to develop good eating habits? In many cases the counselors don't teach those things. It's possible that all you learned was how to lose weight in a boot-camp atmosphere. But since you don't live under the thumb of a drill sergeant out in the real world, you can gain back all the weight you lost.

Ginger, fifteen, lost 22 pounds and was 16 pounds from her goal: I went to the same weight reduction camp for a month every summer for five years in a row. I've had a weight problem all my life and the camp always helped me lose 15 to 20 pounds. But I never felt that I was the one losing the weight. It was more like they (the counselors) were losing it for me. After I got home, I put all the weight back on. I felt like a seesaw. Now I'm losing weight the right way for the first time in my life. I'm making the decisions about what to eat. I'm taking the responsibility. It's a lot harder than losing weight in camp, but it's worth it. This time the weight is staying off.

Not all weight reduction camps are bad. Unfortunately, the good ones are hard to find, so if you are thinking of going to one, check it out thoroughly. Write to the camp director and ask these questions:

- ✔ Are campers taught the basics of good nutrition?
- ✔ Are campers taught good eating habits?
- ✔ How much choice does a camper have in planning his daily activities?
- ✔ What percentage of campers have not gained back any of the weight they lost at camp?

If you are spending your summer vacation at home, be on the alert for the dieter's archenemy—boredom. When you are relaxing at home, you become an easy victim of boredom, which leads to temptation, which leads to eating too much of the wrong kinds of food. You need to stay active, mentally and physically. Join the park district's recreation program, swim daily in the community center pool, play tennis, or earn some spending money by washing cars or mowing lawns or some other part-time business venture. And do your best to follow some regular routine such as eating your meals at roughly the same time each day so you aren't faced with hunger pangs.

In many ways, summer vacation is an excellent time to lose weight. You can devote more time to shedding those pounds through physical activity such as swimming, bicycling, or working out. You should be able to cope more easily because you won't have to deal with the teasing in the classroom or the temptation in the school cafeteria. Also, there is less pressure on you because you don't have to worry about homework. Summer is a happy time, and if you are "up," you automatically do better. What's especially great about dieting over the summer is the grand entrance you can make when you return to school in the fall.

19

COPING AT HOME

Here's a diet fact of life: To succeed, you need the full support of your family. With your parents, brothers, sisters, and close relatives behind you all the way, the likelihood of reaching your goal is great. Here's another diet fact of life: If you don't have the support of your family, you face a difficult time of dieting.

Few young people have reached their weight goal in families that were not supportive. It's just too much to ask a person to stick to a diet in a house where no one cares about nutrition, health, and exercise; where the rest of the family eats huge fat-laced, stomach-bulging dinners; where the pantry is crammed with cookies, cupcakes, and snacks; where the family form of exercising is walking from the couch to the TV and back; where the only love shown in the house is for Mom's cooking. If you are in such a home, you need a triple dose of determination and a remarkably positive attitude to boost you over incredible obstacles.

Even in supportive families, dieters sometimes fall victim because parents, brothers, sisters, and loved ones are human and they make mistakes—sometimes out of love, sometimes out of carelessness. Here are some of the more common diet booby traps at home and ways to avoid them:

The family eats big meals in front of you. One of the toughest things about dieting isn't watching what you eat, it's watching what your family eats. You can't expect your family to change its eating pattern overnight just because you are on a diet. If family members are used to big meals of meat and potatoes and bread and butter, they will probably continue to eat that way. Their actions can turn your dinners into a struggle against temptation, especially when you first start the diet.

It may seem cruel if the family sets out an Italian feast of spaghetti, meatballs, sausage, and garlic bread while you stare at your broiled 3-ounce ground beef patty. How do you avoid this scene? I don't advocate splitting up the family at dinnertime, but if temptation is a problem for you during the early days of the diet, I recommend that you eat elsewhere or at some other time if the family is planning a big special meal. Eat before they do so that by the time dinner rolls around for the rest of the family, your stomach is full and you can join them in table talk without feeling tempted. Or ask the family to eat that big special meal on an evening when you won't be home at dinnertime, because you are spending the night with a friend or are involved in an extracurricular activity at school.

Better yet, try to work out an agreement with them. Ask them to base their dinners around the foods you eat during the first few weeks. They can add sauces and gravies and have more helpings than you if they wish.

For example, let's say you are going to have broiled chicken, green beans, cauliflower, a salad, and a baked apple for dessert. Your family could use those same foods as a basis for their dinner except they could have larger portions of chicken, stuffing, a cheese sauce over their cauliflower, a salad with creamy dressing, and apple pie. The difference between what you eat and what they eat is at least 500 extra calories. This arrangement serves several purposes. First, you are less likely to be bothered by temptation if your family is eating chicken and vegetables just as you are. Second, you buy time. After the first few weeks on the diet, you become accustomed to the new foods and are less likely to want to eat any of the fattening meals that your family prepares. Third, your family may learn to appreciate a healthier way of eating and may actually adopt new eating patterns too.

> *Jason, fourteen, lost 22 pounds and was 13 pounds from his goal:* I didn't receive much support from my family during the first few days on the diet. They kept eating like they did before and teased me about my "diet food." I came back with, "This isn't diet food, this is good food. You should try it because it's healthy and you could all stand to lose a few pounds." I couldn't believe it, but they said they'd try to eat more of the things that I eat and now that's exactly what they do.

The family has a habit of snacking on junk food. Well-meaning family members may applaud you for your dieting efforts and yet not think twice about how they may unknowingly be sabotaging your diet by snacking in front of you. Dad is still going to enjoy his after-dinner ice cream sundae. Mom isn't about to give up her nightly nibble of cheese and crackers. And Sis will always be in front of the TV with her cookies and milk. You don't need to see them packing away all those empty calories. Ask them to help you out by eating their snacks in another room. Or you can leave the room. Maybe your parents could snack to their hearts' content after you have gone to bed. Or (this might be too much to ask, but it's worth a try) request that the family get rid of the junk food in the house. If they yearn for a candy bar or an ice cream cone, they can go out and get it—and eat it there.

Helen, thirteen, lost 18 pounds and was 10 pounds from her goal: I used to bring my dad his beer and peanuts every night when we would watch TV. I always had chips and dip and soda. But after I went on the diet, I gave those things up but my dad sure didn't. He still wanted me to bring him his junk food. I refused. He got mad at me, but I didn't give in. I told him peanuts were for elephants and they were fattening. He didn't like that at all but I notice that he has cut down quite a bit on the peanuts—but not the beer.

Your brothers and sisters deliberately tempt and tease you. We all get into family arguments now and then, and sometimes when you are fighting with a brother or sister, they don't fight fair. The angry words zero in on a sore point—your weight. Or perhaps your little brother, thinking it's fun to tempt you, walks by eating a big piece of fudge and says, "Wouldn't you like to have a bite?" You'd love to shove that candy down his throat. But let's back up a minute to look at ways in which these scenes could be avoided.

Arrange a truce with your brothers and sisters—and even go so far as to put it down in writing. You could work out a deal that you won't poke fun at your brother's acne problem if he lays off the fat jokes and teasing. Or you will let your sister borrow your makeup in exchange for her promise not to eat junk food in front of you. The best approach might be the direct approach. Go up to your brothers and sisters and tell them, "I need your help." Let them feel as though they have a stake in your dieting success. It's to their advantage because they may be feeling some of the fallout from the teasing you receive from others at school or in the neighborhood. They may feel self-conscious about being seen with you in public because you are fat. Actually, most young people in my classes report that their brothers and sisters are very supportive of their dieting efforts.

Carlos, thirteen, lost 23 pounds and was 11 pounds from his goal: I did not get much support from my sisters at first. I was always being teased about being the only fat kid in the family. My sisters used to make big banana splits and eat them in front of me and talk about how delicious they were. I really wanted some, but I wouldn't give in. When my sisters saw how serious I was about dieting, they stopped teasing me and began encouraging me.

Your parents don't give you encouragement. No matter how much responsibility you handle on this diet and how good you feel about yourself as you lose weight, it's still awfully nice to be given a pat on the back once in a while from your parents.

Most parents are full of encouragement. But sometimes, perhaps because of bills or work or personal problems, parents tend to forget to praise their dieting son or daughter for each little success. This could get downright discouraging, especially if you are reaching a difficult time during the diet and you need a little boost. Naturally, if you must beg for compliments, anything your parents say to you may seem insincere. But don't be afraid to remind your parents that you do appreciate and look forward to their kind comments because they help make you feel good. Besides, there might be times when you need one of your parents to talk to when you are feeling low, someone you can confide in, someone who can give you a fresh new perspective to help you cope.

Diana, fifteen, lost 20 pounds and was 12 pounds from her goal: My parents decided to let me handle the diet totally on my own. They didn't want a thing to do with it because they are both very much overweight. After the first month I really wanted some good feedback from them, but I didn't want to come right out and ask because it would be like fishing for compliments. So I started talking to my parents about the diet and explained how it worked and how great I felt. A few days later Mom said she was proud of what I had accomplished so far. And yesterday Dad came back from a long business trip and told me I looked terrific. I told them I needed to hear those kinds of things and I thanked them very much. Those compliments made my day.

Your parents nag you. There's nothing worse than having a parent constantly harp at you about your diet. "Did you drink all your water today?" "Did you eat your three pieces of fruit?" "Make sure you eat all those vegetables on your plate." You can get hounded so much you are ready to chuck the diet just so you don't have to listen to all the nagging.

Politely but firmly put a stop to this with a family meeting. Tell your parents that this is *your* diet and that *you* are in control. Tell them you are following the diet very closely, so nobody has to worry about how much or how little you eat or drink of the proper foods every day. Your parents shouldn't have any reason to badger you because they can soon see the results of the diet for themselves.

If you feel you are being grilled, be understanding. Your parents are probably overly concerned. Give them as many details about your progress as you can without feeling uncomfortable. If they press you for more information, politely tell them something like, "I am doing fine on the diet. I'm happy with myself and I really don't want to talk about it right now. I appreciate your concern. Please try to understand my feelings." In most cases, parents will back off.

Alice, sixteen, lost 17 pounds and was 22 pounds from her goal: My mother begged me to try the diet. I mean begged. She even cried and pleaded with me to lose weight for her. I was shocked. I didn't know my weight was so important to her. So I went on the diet just for her. I quickly discovered that this became her diet, not mine, and she hounded me morning till night, wanting to know every single ounce of food I ate. I got so fed up with her that I threatened to quit. We got into a big fight and then it dawned on me that I had been short-changing myself. I can't diet for someone else. I can only diet for myself. That means I'm responsible and I shouldn't have to answer to anybody but myself. I told my mother that the only way I could lose weight was if she left me alone. Since then there have been no problems.

Tony, fifteen, lost 28 pounds and was 10 pounds from his goal: After the first week of "Don't eat this" and "Don't eat that" and "Eat this" and "Eat that" I set my parents straight. I told them I didn't want them involved in my diet. It's *my* business. I created the problem and I must handle it myself. All I ask from my parents is a nice comment every now and then, and to make sure that I have the food I need in the house. So far they've been pretty good about it.

Your family rewards you with food. Your parents or close relatives may wrongly believe that you suffer on a diet. They feel so sorry for you that they try to sneak you some high-calorie treat as if it were a file baked inside a cake to be smuggled to a prisoner in jail. Your loved ones probably equate love with food. If they think you are unhappy, then that's all the more reason why they want to give you food that is not on the diet.

Or they may offer you a treat as a reward for doing so well on the diet. For example, Johnny has just lost 20 pounds and his father is so proud he decides to reward Johnny by taking him out for a Super Scooper Triple Ripple hot fudge banana split. No way, José! Can you imagine Prince Charming telling Snow White, "Listen, babe, now that you've recovered from that poison apple ordeal, go ahead and sink your teeth into another poison apple." Some treat. If your parents want to give you a treat or reward you for your dieting successes, work out an arrangement whereby the payoff is something other than food. It could be an outing at an amusement park, or a weekend camping trip. Of course, the best reward is looking in the mirror and seeing a slim new figure, a trim new physique.

Craig, twelve, lost 15 pounds and was 6 pounds from his goal: My family is behind me a hundred percent—all eight of them—and to give me an extra push each week, they each chip in one dollar into a pool and I put one buck in too. Then every week that I lose weight, I get to keep the money. If I gain weight, then all the money is given back for that week. So far I've made $60.

Suzanne, fourteen, lost 25 pounds and was 9 pounds from her goal: My parents and I don't believe in rewards. I have to do this for myself. One of the most important things in life is knowing that you can do something good for yourself. I don't need an incentive from anyone else.

Divorced parents don't support the diet. If your parents are divorced and share joint child custody, you probably spend time in the households of both your mother and father. In some cases, this spells trouble because one parent doesn't want to or doesn't know how to support the diet.

For instance, on weekends Sally visits her father, whose kitchen skills stop with pouring milk into a bowl of cereal. He never has the proper food in the refrigerator. So he eats most of his meals at fast food restaurants or pops frozen dinners into the microwave. To stay on the diet, it's up to Sally to prepare the meals. On Friday, she and her dad go shopping for the right foods to last through the weekend. It's the best way to insure that she stays on the diet.

If you are visiting a parent who has remarried or lives out of town, send a copy of the diet in advance and offer to help with the shopping and preparing of the meals.

Whichever divorced parent you visit, he or she undoubtedly wants to show you a good time by taking you to pizza places and the amusement park or the ice cream parlor. You get offered all sorts of food goodies, all of which may taste great but happen to wreck your diet. What do you do? Talk straight with your parent: "I want to be with you and enjoy your company and have fun. That doesn't mean we have to eat things that are not good for me. My diet is very important to me and I want it to be important to you. I need your help and understanding. You can show your love to me by supporting me in my efforts to diet." A bigger problem may develop if the divorce is particularly bitter. One of your parents may simply ignore the diet because he or she doesn't want anything to do with any plan that your other parent supports—whether or not it could benefit you.

In such a case, call up your parent and explain that you will send him or her a copy of the foods you can eat. Ask the parent if there are foods on the list that he or she likes too, and say that you would be glad to help prepare the meals. Try to strike a bargain: "Look, I have been on this diet for several weeks and it's working great. I really feel happy about myself. I'm sure you'll be proud of me too. So could you help me stick to my diet, please?" Your parent will probably go along with your wishes. If your diet is extremely important to you and you aren't getting support, lay it on the line: "If you can't support my efforts to diet, then I'd rather not come to visit you." You should be able to avoid most of these hassles by sitting down with your parents and stepparents separately and explaining what their cooperation means to you and your success.

David, thirteen, lost 27 pounds and was 6 pounds from his goal: I was close to reaching my goal when I visited my mother in another state for three weeks. My stepmother sent my mother a copy of the diet, but when I went to visit, she insisted I eat all the things I used to love and forget about "the stupid diet." She's a great cook and she baked pies and cakes and I just couldn't resist. When I returned home, I had gained six pounds. It was much harder for me to go back on the diet the second time.

Divorce is a traumatic time for everyone and is often one of the reasons why young people gain weight. They are so upset that they find comfort through food or they escape from tension in the house by raiding the refrigerator. If you are caught in the middle of a divorce, perhaps you are better off not trying to go on a diet at this time. Wait until things cool down. With so much turmoil going on, a diet may just be too much for you to deal with. However, many young people in my classes have managed to handle the diet once the divorce became final.

Grandparents and relatives ignore the diet and offer you food. Grandparents and great-grandparents can often innocently wreck your diet. In some cases, the older they are, the harder time they have understanding why you need to diet. That's because they come from a different generation, where overweight meant health and beauty. To them, chubby cheeks are cute; thick arms and legs are signs of sturdiness. Grandmothers often use food as an expression of love. It gives them such pride and pleasure when their grandchildren devour a plateful of homemade cookies. Believe me, it isn't easy to say no when Grandma leads you by the hand into the kitchen and whispers, "I've made these oatmeal cookies just for you. Go ahead, eat as many as you want."

Peter, fourteen, faced a similar situation. Right after he lost 23 pounds on the diet, he visited his grandparents. "Here, have some candy," urged his grandmother, holding a loaded candy jar.

"No, thanks. I can't have any. I'm on a diet."

"It's okay. You've lost enough weight," she insisted.

"I really don't want any candy."

So Grandma left the room and returned with a dinner

plate full of crackers, some topped with peanut butter, others with cheese.

Peter still refused, saying the only thing that worked: "I didn't come here to eat. I came here to see you and Grandpa."

To avoid further confrontations, Peter suggested that his grandparents stock the refrigerator with fresh fruit. That way Grandma could still derive some pleasure in offering food without destroying Peter's diet.

If you are going to your grandmother's house, give her a list of foods you can have ahead of time, or better yet go shopping with her. Help prepare the meals at her house and explain in detail exactly what the diet is and why it is necessary for you to lose weight.

It's possible that you may get caught in the middle of an argument between your parents, who defend your diet, and your grandparents, who don't. The scene can get pretty ugly. One way to avoid this situation is to invite your grandparents over to your house, where you feel more in control of what you can and cannot eat. Take the heat off your parents by explaining to your grandparents that dieting is your idea and you are losing weight to improve yourself. Then serve your grandparents the same dinner that you eat so they can see how nutritious, filling, and delicious it is.

> *Christie, thirteen, lost 22 pounds and was 10 pounds from her goal:* Every time I went over to Grandma's house, she had a cake waiting for me. She'd say, "Go ahead and enjoy it. I baked it just for you." I'd say, "I can't have it because I'm on a diet." Then she'd get angry and start scolding Mom for getting me to go on the diet. She'd say I didn't need a diet. There's always so much tension in her house that I can't stand it. Everyone always gets mad, so I told her that I'm not going to visit her anymore until I reach my goal. And I haven't.

Elyse, thirteen, lost 18 pounds and was 10 pounds from her goal: I have grandparents who just didn't believe that a kid should diet. When I went on the diet, they invited me over to their house all the time. They live only a few blocks away. Every time I went over there, they tried to bribe me to eat, and promised to take me to the movies if I'd eat a big dinner with them. They were always putting down the diet. One day I couldn't stand it anymore and I started to cry. I told them how awful it is to be a fat kid and that I wanted to lose weight and be thin. For the first time they understood me and why I had to go on a diet and stick with it. Now I go over to their house more often. We do lots of things together like walking, bike riding, taking nature walks, and gardening. Best of all, they buy me an outfit with every 10 pounds I lose.

If your relatives persist to the point where they won't take no for an answer, that's the time to get tough. Be firm without hurting their feelings. Rather than lashing out at their actions, explain the importance of not straying from your diet. You should be able to convince them.

Because it is so important to have the support of your family throughout your diet, take the time and make the effort to gain the assistance and understanding of loved ones. With their support, your chances of reaching your goal are much greater.

Greg, fourteen, lost 16 pounds and was 6 pounds from his goal: I just returned from my uncle's farm where I spent a month and had a great time. All the relatives were complimenting me on my weight and they encouraged me to follow the diet. We came up with different recipes for the fresh vegetables that we picked from the garden and we ate cheese and drank skim milk from their dairy plant. I came home eight pounds lighter.

20

OOPS!

You might make it through the diet without a single mistake. But I doubt it. After all, human beings make mistakes. Occasionally, some of the kids in my diet classes have what I call an "oops." They eat something they know they shouldn't.

We don't use the word "cheat" in class because it means being dishonest. If you start thinking that you are a cheater for what you did, then you might start calling yourself other bad names, and before you know it, you could tumble into the pit of low self-esteem. People with low self-esteem do not do well on this diet because they think, "What's the use?" Then they begin to eat—and eat.

That's why I use the word "oops." When you munch on a bag of corn chips or eat a scoop of ice cream, it's nothing more than a simple mistake—an oops. It's sort of like misspelling a word on a test. Perhaps you knew how to spell the word but you were in a hurry and you accidentally switched two letters and got it wrong. It was a simple mistake.

If you have an oops on the diet, stay cool. Recognize what you did and then forget about it. Get right back on the diet. Follow the example of major league baseball players. There isn't a superstar on the field who hasn't committed an error by dropping a fly ball or throwing the ball wildly past the first baseman. But the players don't quit. They know that errors are part of the game. They put their mistakes behind them and go on playing as hard as they can.

Rona, fifteen, lost 16 pounds and was 15 pounds from her goal: I messed up a couple of weeks ago. There was a bake sale at school. I couldn't help it. I bought a couple of brownies and ate them. I kept thinking, "I don't care. I want them and I'm going to eat them. So I'll be fat." I put the diet way in the back of my mind. But after I ate them, I felt really depressed and got mad at myself for messing up. I went on a weekend eating binge. It was like another person eating all that food, not me. I gained a couple of pounds and that made me even more angry with myself. I've built up a lot of negative feelings toward my mistakes and that hasn't helped me on my diet. I often wonder why I am drawn to food so much, but the answer lies within myself. I'm very aware of what I am doing wrong and I am still working on sticking to the diet.

Craig, twelve, lost 15 pounds and was 6 pounds from his goal: When I go off the diet, I figure, "Well, I've already screwed up so another one or two pieces of cake won't matter." When my dad catches me and scolds me, I find myself eating and eating just to get even with him. Then I feel real guilty and promise myself never to do it again. Except I can't help myself and I have another piece of cake.

Rona and Craig will continue to have trouble because they are stuck in a rut of guilt, anger, and surrender—three diet wreckers. These young people dwell on their past failures rather than march forward on the diet with the determination to succeed. How can they possibly reward themselves with slim new bodies at the end of the diet if they constantly punish themselves with food binges and bad feelings?

An oops is not worth all this emotional garbage. It's not as if you've committed some horrible crime that will put you behind bars for the rest of your life. When you have an oops, spend a minute thinking positive thoughts. Look back at all the weight you have managed to lose so far. You've proven to yourself you can lose weight.

Carlos, thirteen, lost 23 pounds and was 11 pounds from his goal: I know what I'm supposed to eat on this diet, and when I fall off, it makes me feel bad that sometimes I just can't say no to some food. But I shake it off right away. I think back to all the times when I could have gone off the diet but didn't. I won't give in to bad thoughts about myself because I believe in what I'm doing. I have faith in myself.

One of the most important pieces of advice that I can give you about an oops is to pick up the diet where you left off—as if nothing had happened. Some dieters who commit an oops and eat too much try to starve themselves the next few days to make up for their oops. Don't try it. You usually do much more harm than good that way. Not eating could throw your body out of whack, deprive you of needed nutrients, and leave you open to extreme swings of mood from being happy one minute to suddenly feeling sad the next. If you feel you absolutely must do something to counteract your oops, then jog longer than usual, bicycle harder, or do some other physical activity. You probably won't burn off all the extra calories you added, but it can make you feel better. The worst thing that might happen as a result of an oops is that you might not lose weight that week. In that case, you probably will lose weight the following week. Trying too hard to counteract your oops can lead to serious health problems.

Marsha, sixteen, lost 20 pounds and was 22 pounds from her goal: Last week I broke down and had a piece of pie. Then I had another and a third piece. It was a bummer, a downer. No one could say anything to make me feel better. It was as if the food won and I lost. But then I thought I'd be smart and beat this oops. So I swallowed two laxatives that night, hoping to clean out my system. Well, about two in the morning I woke up with severe cramps and diarrhea. I felt sick all the next day. I'll never try that stunt again.

Even if you find that you can get away with having one little oops one week without gaining any weight, don't "accidentally" plan on having any more. If you do . . . SURPRISE! . . . you are going to gain weight.

Jeff, fifteen, lost 25 pounds and reached his goal: I was going great guns on the diet and sometime during the second month I ate two cupcakes. I still lost weight that week. That was like a green flag to me because I had another seven oopses over the next three weeks. Only this time I didn't get away with it. I gained two pounds. I thought, "Man, are you dumb. You can't be on half of a diet. You either stick to it or get off it." I learned the only way you can lose weight is if you follow the diet.

When an oops occurs, don't look for someone else to blame. You could have had an oops for a variety of reasons—someone upset you, someone tempted you, or you were bored. Searching for blame is a negative activity that serves no useful purpose. In fact, it can lead to more hassles, like triggering an argument with a friend or loved one. You have better things to do with your time.

Peter, fourteen, lost 46 pounds and reached his goal: I was with some friends and we went into the 7-Eleven store and they bought ice cream sandwiches. They were saying how good the ice cream sandwiches tasted and I just caved in and bought one too and ate it. Afterward, I felt angry at myself, but I took it out on them and accused them of deliberately tempting me. I told them they were lousy friends. That night it dawned on me that nobody's perfect and that it's up to me to follow the diet. I talked it over with my friends the next day and asked for their help. After that, I never let an oops bother me.

If it makes you feel better, go ahead and talk about your oops with someone you trust. But to be honest with you, you are probably better off just putting it all behind you and going ahead with your daily life and the diet.

Debbie, fourteen, lost 31 pounds and was 16 pounds from her goal: Once I eat something I shouldn't have, I get guilt feelings and think the diet isn't worth it. The only thoughts I have are that everything is going wrong in my life. But having a close friend that I can confide in helps me through the rough spots. She gets me to see things in a different way. She talks about the day when I will reach my goal and how great I'll feel. I need that sometimes.

I can't stress enough the need for positive thoughts, especially right after you have an oops. Okay, you goofed. So promise to try a little harder the next time.

Heidi, thirteen, lost 24 pounds and was 11 pounds from her goal: When I have an oops—which doesn't happen very often—it's always over something I really enjoyed eating. I know it's wrong and I don't mope or pout over it. I don't forget it either. I just get right back on the diet because I have a lot of confidence in myself to reach my goal. I just keep trying my best.

Reaching Your Goal and Staying There

21

THE BIG MOMENT

As you step on the scale, your heart pounds with anticipation. This could be the moment, the one big moment for which you've worked so hard. You hold your breath and look down at the scale, staring at it until you are sure your eyes are not playing some sort of trick. There is no mistake. The scale shows a number that has special meaning only to you, a number that has stayed locked in your brain since the day you first started the diet. You look at the number for a long time. A warm glowing feeling begins flowing through your veins. You did it! You have finally reached your goal!

This is a magic moment, one to be cherished because it is dramatic proof that you have "the right stuff." You have taken responsibility, shown determination, and managed to cope. You have battled temptation and teasing—and won. And now all the hard work—planning menus, preparing meals, learning new eating habits, sticking to the diet—has paid off.

You feel wonderful. And why shouldn't you? You have accomplished a very difficult task. And you did it on your own. More important, you did it for yourself.

Kevin, twelve, lost 24 pounds and reached his goal: When I reached my goal, I was so happy. I had not done anything before that had made me feel as good as this. For two days, I felt fantastic. My parents celebrated by taking me out to buy some clothes, and for once I really enjoyed shopping. It sure was different from the time I was chubby and nothing fit me like it should. Now that I'm at my goal, I don't think about running out and eating something new. I'm not going to goof up now—not after I've worked so hard to look like this.

Thomas, thirteen, lost 44 pounds and reached his goal: I hit my goal about a week before our big family reunion at our house. Would you believe that hardly anyone knew who I was at first? My aunt and uncle thought I was the neighborhood kid. I asked them, "How do you like your new nephew?" I was the talk of the reunion . . . and I loved every minute of it.

Joan, fourteen, lost 50 pounds and reached her goal: I am so happy about what I have done. I feel like a different person, like this isn't really my body, that it's someone else who is thin. It's hard for me to believe it's really me. The biggest shock is to see a picture of me now and compare it with a year ago. I have such mixed feelings. On one hand, I'm embarrassed to think that I looked so fat and ugly. On the other hand, I'm very proud that I've accomplished so much to be the person I am now.

Marsha, sixteen, lost 42 pounds and reached her goal: When I reached my goal, I didn't celebrate or anything like that. Instead I sat down and thought about how much I had changed. I used to be shy because I thought that people were just going to laugh in my face. I had no social life or dates. When I went on the diet I kept wondering if it was all worth it. I had my share of oopses and low points and thought that it would take forever to reach my goal. But I stayed with the diet and now I feel so good about myself. I like the way I look. My life has certainly changed for the better. One of the best things that has happened to me is that I'm dating a real nice guy and we're going to homecoming this year. It'll be the first time I've ever gone to a dance with a date.

Eric, twelve, lost 27 pounds and reached his goal: I only did one thing different than usual on the day I reached my goal. There's a tree in the park about a block from my house that all the kids in the neighborhood like to climb. I couldn't get up it when I was fat, and I got teased. One of my goals was to climb the tree and I decided to do it on the day I hit my weight goal. So that's what I did.

Lauren, fifteen, lost 25 pounds and reached her goal: My best friend and I have the same body build and are the same height. Before I started the diet, I weighed 25 pounds more than she did. I wore a size 38 blouse and she wore a size 32. She said it would be great if we were the same weight so then we could wear each other's clothes. Well, when I reached my goal, I went over to her house and went into her closet and pulled out one of her blouses that I had always admired and put it on. That was my way of telling her I'd reached my goal.

Christie, thirteen, lost 42 pounds and reached her goal: My dad lives in New York and I kept my diet a secret from him. I didn't want to visit him until I lost all that weight. When I hit my goal, I flew to New York. I got off the plane and he looked right past me. He didn't recognize me—and I was standing right in front of him. When I said, "Hi, Daddy!" he couldn't believe it. He was so proud of me.

Sarah, fourteen, lost 31 pounds and reached her goal: Right after I hit my goal, I had a magic moment. It happened during church. The minister welcomes new people to the congregation during services and on this day he made a special announcement. He said a member of the congregation had lost so much weight that she was considered a new person. It was me he was talking about. He had me stand up and the whole church clapped.

Not everybody gets so charged up on the actual day they reach their goal. The reason is simple. They were losing weight steadily throughout the diet and were receiving compliments and adjusting to their slimmer way of life. By the time they hit their goal, it was sort of anticlimactic. They were already enjoying their new life weeks before they reached the magic number.

Terri, sixteen, lost 53 pounds and reached her goal: The big moment for me happened about the third month on the diet when I returned to school in the fall. I had lost about 30 pounds and some of the people who hadn't seen me through the summer could really tell the difference. Also, I had a tremendous sense of being in control. When you finally separate yourself from eating all the time, it's a feeling of freedom, like the first Monday after school lets out for the summer. It's great, especially when I can feel bones in my body that I never felt before. That's better than any glazed doughnut I ever ate.

It's okay to toot your horn a little bit when you reach your goal. Be proud of your accomplishment. An eighth grader in one of my classes used himself as a subject for his school science fair project. He drew up a chart showing how much he weighed before and after the diet and how many calories he consumed daily. He gave a demonstration of what a calorie is (a unit of energy in food, remember?) and also included before and after pictures of himself.

When you reach your goal, you may be anxious to tell

others who are overweight how effective the diet is. Be careful what you say. It's one thing to answer questions for someone who is interested, but it's another thing to preach or nag. Let's say your friend could afford to lose 30 pounds. If you get on his back for eating junk food, fries, and colas, you are asking for trouble—and may lose a friend. No matter how much you may want to help your friend, think back to when you were fat. How did you want to be approached so you weren't embarrassed? You probably wanted to be the one to bring up the subject rather than having someone else remind you how fat you were. One of the biggest turnoffs is the person who brags about his weight loss and goes up to a fat person and says, "You're fat, but you don't have to be anymore if you do what I did." A much better approach to an overweight friend might be: "I'm really happy with my weight loss. If you'd like to know more about how I lost weight, I'd be glad to tell you." Remember, this diet works only for those who are ready to make a commitment.

Reaching your goal does not automatically guarantee you a fantastic school life of friends, straight A's, dates, and star status on the basketball team. However, when you hit your weight goal, you are no longer handicapped socially, physically, or psychologically by being fat. Freed from the shackles of an overweight body, you can take advantage of so many more opportunities. Since you have proven to yourself that you possess the determination to succeed, set your sights on other goals. Understand that achievements are reached by hard work. Whether you want to be a dancer or a third baseman, you must practice, practice, practice to develop your talents. Success won't happen just because you are now thin.

Some young people who reach their goals think they will become instantly popular. Don't make the same mistake in wishful thinking. If you were fat and inconsiderate before you went on the diet and haven't changed your personality, then people aren't going to like you no matter how much weight you've lost. The only difference is that now you are slim and inconsiderate.

Look upstairs in your head and decide to be the person you want to be. Now that you have lost all that weight, take full advantage of the situation in your personal life and in your career goals. Keep in mind that the doors to opportunity are not going to open automatically because you hit your goal. However, these doors aren't going to be slammed in your face as they may have been in the past when you were fat. You still must make the effort to open those doors and step right in.

Sometimes reaching their goal can lead to very serious problems for young people who never grasped the importance of remaining in total control of a healthy, nutritious eating plan. There is an old saying: You can never be too rich or too thin. I don't care to comment on the first part of the sentence, but to the last half, I say WRONG! You *can* be too thin.

Some young people, usually girls, simply don't know when to stop dieting. They are victims of a disease known as anorexia nervosa, a severe illness that afflicts thousands of young people.

In the early stages of anorexia nervosa, the victim may feel fine and look terrific, but she is not satisfied by her weight loss or the appearance of her body. Even after she has hit her goal, she is obsessed with the need to lose still more weight. She begins to overexercise and seldom eats, even to the point where she is literally starving herself.

Her hair begins to fall out and she ceases to menstruate. Because she is not consuming enough food to meet her body's energy demands, her body draws on muscles for energy. As a result, her muscles become smaller and less efficient and more easily fatigued. She develops dry skin, has trouble sleeping, and notices that small cuts heal slowly. In the advanced stages of the illness, she could suffer convulsions, heart failure—even death.

Fortunately, this disease can be successfully treated with both medical and psychological care. This is not something that can be treated solely by the victim or her parents. The sooner she seeks professional help, the sooner she is likely to recover.

Occasionally I meet a young person who mistakenly thinks that once he attains his weight goal, he can go out and eat anything he wants. Then there is the young person who tries to lose an extra five pounds below his weight goal so he can go out and enjoy all the things that he had deprived himself of during the diet. It's a shame, because these young people haven't learned very much about nutrition or good eating habits. They haven't understood that they are condemning themselves to a yo-yo life of fat, thin, fat, thin, fat. There is no way they can eat too much of the wrong foods and expect to maintain their ideal weight. They put on five pounds, then another five pounds, and end up fat again. It's back on another diet.

> *Mardee, fourteen, lost 26 pounds and reached her goal:* It took me two times on the diet to get it right. The first time around it was more or less a game to me. I didn't do it for myself. I lost weight because my parents insisted. They were always on my case so I stuck to the diet pretty much and lost 20 pounds. I was so happy I went straight to an ice cream shop and ordered a gigantic banana split. The next day I had a couple of burgers, fries, and a shake. I went on an eating rampage that didn't end until I had gained back the 20 pounds plus an additional 6. My parents were fit to be tied. I guess I didn't want to learn a thing during the diet. But I wised up the second time around. When I hit my goal again, I knew that I could not go out and eat all the things that had made me fat in the first place.

Controlling your weight is a lifelong responsibility. This doesn't mean you must diet forever. Nor does it mean you can never eat certain foods again. To stay slim and healthy, you must follow a simple but effective maintenance plan.

22

MAINTAINING YOUR IDEAL WEIGHT

Having reached your goal, you are slim—and you want to stay that way.

That means you must follow a maintenance program. This is not a diet but a sensible eating guide for the rest of your life. There's no need to groan. Controlling your weight is a lifetime responsibility, not a lifetime chore. It's really not so difficult, because by the time you reach your goal, eating properly has become second nature to you. You certainly know what is and what isn't good for your health and your weight. So combine your new-found knowledge with the suggestions in this chapter to create your own personal maintenance program.

Let's make one thing clear: Since you may still be growing, maintenance does not necessarily mean that you must stay at your goal weight. It means you must maintain *control* of your weight. Your weight may have to increase gradually to keep up with your height. The correct weight for your height is known as your *ideal weight*. However, if you have finished growing, then you should keep your goal weight pretty much the same.

Going from a reducing diet to a maintenance program

requires some thought and planning. You can't suddenly start eating anything you want or as much as you want—unless you wish to be fat again. Basically, you should gradually increase the portions of what you eat, eat a wider variety of foods, eat in moderation, and follow a fitness program. Also, by trial and error, you should determine how much food (or, more specifically, how many calories) your body requires to maintain control of your weight.

To put it simply, you can continue eating pretty much the same way you did on the reducing diet, except that you can eat slightly larger quantities and have a bigger selection of foods to choose from. But don't kid yourself. It's still thumbs down on the foods that made you fat. Before these points are discussed in detail, you need a better picture of what to eat when going from the reducing diet to a maintenance program.

What to Eat

As I mentioned in chapter 3, "Why You Are Fat," you need about fifty nutrients, including vitamins and minerals, to stay healthy. These nutrients are in the foods you normally eat. Since no single food supplies all the essential nutrients, you should eat a variety of foods so you won't suffer from a deficiency of any particular nutrient.

Gradually introduce new foods from the four basic food groups. As you recall, the food in the reducing diet came from these food groups. Now you can add more varieties from these groups. For example:

✔ *Fruits and vegetables*: starchy vegetables such as chick-peas (also called garbanzos), corn, lima beans, mashed potatoes, navy beans, peas, sweet potatoes, winter squash, yams, avocado, dates, figs, raisins.

- ✔ *Grain and fiber*: bagels, biscuits, corn bread, corn muffins, crackers, English muffins, grits, macaroni, noodles, rice, spaghetti.
- ✔ *Dairy*: cream cheese, ice milk, ice cream, milk custards, milk puddings, other cheeses, sour cream, low-fat flavored yogurt, frozen yogurt.
- ✔ *Protein-rich foods*: bacon, beef tacos, brisket, chili, corned beef, luncheon meats, spare ribs, peanut butter, nuts, dried beans.

Don't add too many new food items on your maintenance plan on any one day because then you risk consuming too many calories. For example, don't have pancakes for breakfast, a peanut butter and jelly sandwich for lunch, and spaghetti and meatballs for dinner all in the same day. Space the new foods out throughout the week, as shown in the sample maintenance menu (see pages 217–224).

If you wish, you can add a little more pizzazz to your meals with moderate amounts of sauces and gravies. But be careful, because they are loaded with calories and notorious for adding extra pounds in a hurry.

Cook foods with little or no added fat. Meat and poultry should be trimmed of visible fat and braised, broiled, roasted, baked, or cooked over a charcoal grill. Fish should be baked or broiled, while vegetables should be steamed, baked, boiled, or stir-fried in a wok. Meat, fish, and poultry should be lean.

You should continue drinking three glasses of low-fat milk, especially acidophilus, to help give strength and structure to bones and teeth. Continue drinking plenty of other liquids, especially water, as well.

How to Eat

On a maintenance program, you can eat portions slightly larger than those on the reducing diet. Instead of a three-ounce steak with dinner, make it four ounces. (Under certain conditions discussed later in this chapter it might be possible to eat even bigger portions.)

Naturally, the key word here is moderation. As you introduce new foods to your menu, eat limited portions, certainly no larger than those on the reducing diet. To some young people, the tendency is to load up on a favorite food such as spaghetti and ignore other good food.

Don't forget to continue your good eating habits. Eat slowly, eat three meals a day, eat only in the dining room or kitchen, eat without distractions and . . . well . . . you should know the rest. If you need a refresher, look back at chapter 10, "The Good Eating Habit."

What to Avoid

There may be times when you will want to eat junk food. Do your best to make these moments few and far between or you will see the difference when you step on the scale. Fortunately, what you'll probably discover is that you no longer have a craving for these foods or that you actually find them distasteful.

Do your best to avoid the following:

- ✘ *Junk food snacks*. These include things that are sweet and gooey, like candy; smooth and thick, like cream-filled cookies; and greasy-crisp, like potato chips or corn chips. Also try to avoid sodas. Instead, continue to eat and drink nutritious snacks such as raw fruit and vegetables, fruit juice, tomato juice, V-8, club soda with lemon.
- ✘ *Foods high in fat*. Avoid butter, cream, shortenings, and also deep-fried foods, which are high in calories because fat is absorbed during cooking.
- ✘ *Sugar and sweets*. Whether or not you are on a diet, too much sugar is harmful because it leads to tooth decay

and has no nutritional value. It can produce psychological dependence bordering on addiction. The more you eat, the more you want. Limit your intake of refined white sugar, brown sugar, honey, syrups, jams, jellies, marmalade, candy, soft drinks, cakes, and cookies. Sugar goes under other names as well, so check labels for corn syrup, dextrose, fructose, glucose, and lactose. If you need a sweetener, use fresh fruit, Equal, or a NutraSweet product.

✘ *Salt.* You really don't need to use the salt from the shaker because many foods contain "hidden" sodium, especially instant foods, canned foods, luncheon meats, condiments, salty snacks, cured meats, beverages, and pickled foods. Try to stay away from these convenience foods as much as you can. If you must flavor your food, use low-sodium salt or better yet use spices such as pepper.

Determining How Much to Eat

How much can you eat, or in other words, how many calories can you consume and still maintain control of your weight? Sorry, there is no easy answer. This is something you must find out for yourself. Your age, sex, bone structure, metabolism, and the amount of physical activity you engage in all play a role in your daily calorie requirements.

The best way to figure out how much you can eat is the trial and error method. It may take several weeks before you find an answer. To help you, follow the sample seven-day maintenance menu (beginning on page 217) for one week. The daily menus average about 2,100 calories, which is about 600 calories more than the daily menus on the reducing diet. At the end of the week, weigh yourself. If you lose weight, that means your body requires more calories, so you should increase your consumption of food to a moderate degree. If you gain weight, then cut back on the amount of food. Once you reach two weeks in a row in which you have not gained or lost, then assume you are consuming the right amount of calories and the proper amount of food.

Continue to weigh yourself weekly so you can stay in tune with your body and make any adjustments necessary to maintain control of your weight. If you experience difficulty in controlling your weight, take time to reflect on what you might be doing wrong: Are you simply eating too much? Are you not exercising enough? Are you returning to bad eating habits? Are you eating the wrong foods? By all means, go back to the reducing diet until you have regained control of your weight and are back to your ideal weight.

The more active you are, the more you can eat without gaining weight because you are burning up calories. However, if you reduce the amount of physical activity you engage in weekly, you must also cut back on your food consumption or risk increasing your weight again.

Adjusting Your Ideal Weight

There is nothing wrong with gaining weight if you are still growing—provided that your weight is compatible with your height. After you reach your goal, your ideal weight increases with every inch you grow.

You can get a general idea of how much weight you should be gaining while growing. First, you need to keep close tabs on your body's growth, so weigh yourself weekly and measure your height monthly. Armed with these figures, turn to the growth charts on pages 57–60 and plot your height and weight on the graph. Generally speaking, both your height and weight should fall fairly close to the same percentiles. For example, a sixteen-year-old girl who is sixty-two inches tall is in the twenty-fifth percentile, so her weight should probably be somewhere near the twenty-fifth percentile also, at about 110 pounds.

To determine your adjusted ideal weight as you grow, first find the percentile closest to your height on the height-for-age chart. To do this, find your height on the scale at the left of the chart and draw a line across the chart. Where that line intersects your age line, mark an x with a pencil. The curved line closest to your mark is the percentile.

Next, turn to the weight-for-age chart. Find your age at the bottom of the chart and draw a line up to the top of the chart. Where the line intersects the same percentile as that of your height, mark an x with a pencil. Draw a horizontal line from the mark to the weight scale at the left of the chart. The point where the line intersects the weight scale tells you your adjusted ideal weight.

To illustrate, let's look at the growth rate of fourteen-year-old Jason. When he reached his goal, he was sixty-four inches tall and weighed 112 pounds. According to the growth charts, his weight and height were in the fiftieth percentile. In other words, he was the average height and weight for boys his age. As he grows, his height and weight should stay pretty close to the fiftieth percentile. Projecting his growth for the coming year, he should grow three inches (to sixty-seven inches) and gain 14 pounds (to 126 pounds) which are the height and weight for a fifteen-year-old in the fiftieth percentile. That means he can average about a pound per month increase in weight without worrying that he's putting on too much weight. In fact, he's staying well within the boundaries of his adjusted ideal weight as he grows.

It's not as confusing as it sounds. If you have trouble trying to figure out the charts, don't despair. These charts should be used only as a broad, general guide. It's best to consult your doctor to help you find the right weight for you as you grow.

If you experience a major growth spurt of three or four inches, and your ideal adjusted weight is from 10 to 15 pounds higher than your goal weight, don't feel you must put on the extra weight right away by overeating. Continue to eat the proper foods, increasing your portions, and in time you will reach the best weight for you.

Maintain Your Own Fitness Program

Engaging in some type of regular, planned physical activity is just as important on maintenance as it was on the diet. Follow the same fitness plan you had on the reducing diet. Or try to develop a new skill in at least one sport or activity. You don't have to excel in it, just participate enough to gain a sense of accomplishment. It doesn't have to be a competitive team sport. Just work up a sweat and have fun. Try tennis, skiing, ice skating, roller skating, surfing, power lifting, ballet, bicycling, tap dancing.

Even if you don't want to participate in a sport, at least spend thirty minutes a day four or more times a week in some form of vigorous physical activity such as aerobics, jazzercise, brisk walking, swimming, jogging, or doing an exercise routine.

A regular fitness program increases your endurance and coordination. Also, it reduces fatigue, stress, and physical and mental tension. When you are physically active, your heartbeat becomes stronger and circulation improves. As a result, you gain more energy. Furthermore, by using your muscles and joints, you become stronger and more flexible. This improves your posture and your personal appearance. Another benefit of fitness is simply that you feel better and look better. And you reduce the chances of ever becoming fat again.

The maintenance plan, from the menus to the fitness program, makes up a blueprint for creating a healthy, enjoyable, slim life.

Javier, seventeen, lost 46 pounds and has been at his goal for three years: Four years ago when I was still fat, there was no way you could get me to do a lick of exercise. For the last few years since I've been on maintenance, I've been pumping iron and I love it. I'm really into health and nutrition and fitness because I'm proof of what they can do to make you look and feel better. You couldn't get me to go back to my old ways of eating and not exercising for a million bucks.

Tony, fifteen, lost 38 pounds and has been at his goal for two years: The maintenance is easy for me. To tell the truth, I just don't think about food like I used to. When I was fat, all I cared about was food. But it's not that important to me. I'm so used to eating good things that it doesn't bother me in the least to avoid junk food. I can go to Burger King and order a hamburger and iced tea while my friends eat a Whopper, fries, and a soda. Maintenance has just become a way of life. It's no big deal for me.

Helen, thirteen, lost 18 pounds and has been at her goal for one year: The hardest part of maintenance to me is just reminding myself what I should be eating. When you are no longer on a diet, you sometimes forget what you are doing and you end up eating foods you shouldn't have. My stomach has a good memory, and when I eat something bad for me, it lets me know. I just have to pay more attention to what I eat and not get too careless.

The maintenance program is a guide to help keep you from ever suffering a weight problem again. However, don't let it dominate your life or your thoughts. Just be aware of how and what you eat, and stay active. Once you are slim, focus your attention on doing all the things that can make your life terrific.

23

SEVEN-DAY SAMPLE MAINTENANCE MENU

Now that you know what foods you should eat to maintain control of your weight, I want to show you how to arrange them into a nutritional, well-balanced eating plan.

As you study the seven-day sample maintenance menu, you will notice that it contains many of the foods that you've been eating on the reducing diet. There is a reason for this. The foods on the diet are healthy foods—and you should continue to eat them. The basic difference is that on the maintenance program, you can eat slightly larger portions and choose from a wider variety of foods.

Keep in mind that the sample menu can be modified to suit your own preference and needs, as long as you continue to follow the maintenance guidelines. Here is the seven-day sample maintenance menu:

DAY 1 *Thursday*

BREAKFAST

1 serving Rice Krispies
1 cup acidophilus low-fat milk
1 medium peach, sliced
1 slice whole wheat toast, with
    1 teaspoon reduced-calorie soft margarine
4 ounces unsweetened grape juice

LUNCH

1 chicken salad sandwich, made with
    4 ounces skinless cooked chicken breast, diced
    ¼ cup chopped celery
    2 tablespoons mayonnaise
    ½ medium tomato, sliced
    ½ cup shredded lettuce
    1 medium pita bread
1 medium raw carrot, cut into sticks
15 large (or 25 small) cherries
Beverage

DINNER

4 ounces broiled steak, lean only
½ cup Seasoned Mushrooms (see recipe)
1 medium baked potato, with
    1 teaspoon reduced-calorie soft margarine
    1 tablespoon sour cream
1 cup cooked spinach, fresh or frozen, with
    1 teaspoon reduced-calorie soft margarine
2 cups tossed garden salad, with
    2 tablespoons reduced-calorie salad dressing
½ cup chocolate pudding
1 cup acidophilus low-fat milk

SNACKS

2 cups popped popcorn
1 medium orange
1 Piña Colada Milkshake (see recipe)

DAY 2 **Friday**

BREAKFAST

1 cup cooked oatmeal
1 cup acidophilus low-fat milk
One 1½-ounce box raisins
1 slice whole wheat cinnamon toast, with
 1 teaspoon reduced-calorie soft margarine
4 ounces unsweetened grapefruit juice

LUNCH

1 peanut butter and jelly sandwich made with
 2 tablespoons peanut butter
 1 tablespoon jelly
 2 slices whole wheat bread
1 stalk celery, cut into sticks
½ medium cucumber, cut into spears
1 small banana
Beverage

DINNER

4 ounces Broiled Fish Fillet (see recipe), with
 1 tablespoon tartar sauce
½ cup macaroni and cheese
1 cup cooked green beans, fresh or frozen, with
 1 teaspoon reduced-calorie soft margarine
2 cups garden salad, with
 2 tablespoons reduced-calorie dressing
1 cup Frozen Grapes (see recipe)
1 cup acidophilus low-fat milk

SNACKS

2 cups popped popcorn
2 medium plums
1 vanilla milkshake (see Milkshake Marvel recipe)

DAY 3 Saturday

BREAKFAST

2 slices Whole Wheat French Toast (see recipe), with
    1 serving Cinnamon-Margarine Topping (see recipe)
1 cup fresh blackberries
4 ounces orange juice
1 cup acidophilus low-fat milk

LUNCH

1 turkey sandwich, made with
    4 ounces skinless cooked turkey breast, sliced
    2 tablespoons mayonnaise
    lettuce
    ½ medium tomato, sliced
    1 medium pita bread
½ medium green pepper, sliced
6 radishes
2-inch wedge honeydew melon
Beverage

DINNER

4 ounces roast beef, lean only
½ cup mashed potato, with
    2 tablespoons gravy
1 cup cooked fresh or frozen broccoli, with
    1 teaspoon reduced-calorie soft margarine
2 cups tossed garden salad, with
    2 tablespoons reduced-calorie salad dressing
1 cup acidophilus low-fat milk

SNACKS

2 cups popped popcorn
1 medium nectarine
1 raspberry milkshake (see Fruity Milkshake recipe)

SEVEN-DAY SAMPLE MAINTENANCE MENU

DAY 4 **Sunday**

BREAKFAST

1 large egg, any style
2 slices lean bacon, well drained
1 slice whole wheat toast, with
    1 teaspoon reduced-calorie soft margarine
½ fresh medium grapefruit
4 ounces unsweetened apple juice
1 cup hot chocolate, made with
    1 cup acidophilus low-fat milk
    1 teaspoon chocolate flavor mix sweetened with NutraSweet

LUNCH

1 grilled cheese sandwich, made with
    2 slices (2 ounces) American cheese
    2 slices whole wheat bread
    1 teaspoon reduced-calorie soft margarine
1 cup tomato soup (made with milk or water)
1 cup raw cauliflower
1 tablespoon unsalted dry-roasted peanuts
1 medium pear
Beverage

DINNER

4 ounces barbecued skinless chicken breast, with
    2 tablespoons barbecue sauce
1 ear corn on the cob, with
    1 teaspoon reduced-calorie soft margarine
1 cup cole slaw
2 cups watermelon cubes
1 cup acidophilus low-fat milk

SNACKS

2 cups popped popcorn
1 large tangerine
1 almond milkshake (see Milkshake Marvel recipe)

DAY 5 **Monday**

BREAKFAST

⅔ cup cooked enriched farina
1 cup acidophilus low-fat milk
¼ small cantaloupe
1 slice whole wheat toast, with
    1 teaspoon reduced-calorie soft margarine
4 ounces V-8 juice

LUNCH

1 ham sandwich, made with
    3 ounces baked or boiled ham, lean only
    lettuce
    ½ teaspoon mustard
    2 slices whole wheat bread
1 medium raw carrot, cut into sticks
1 stalk celery, cut into sticks
1 cup grapes
Beverage

DINNER

1 serving spaghetti and meatballs, made with
    1½ cups cooked spaghetti
    ½ cup spaghetti sauce
    three 1-ounce meatballs
    2 tablespoons Parmesan cheese
1 medium slice Italian bread, with
    1 teaspoon reduced-calorie soft margarine and
    dash of garlic powder
2 cups tossed garden salad, with
    2 tablespoons reduced-calorie salad dressing
½ cup lime-flavored gelatin, with
    1 medium peach, sliced
1 cup acidophilus low-fat milk

SNACKS

2 cups popped popcorn
One 1½-ounce box raisins
1 Coffee Milkshake (see recipe)

DAY 6 Tuesday

BREAKFAST

1 serving 40% Bran Flakes
1 cup acidophilus low-fat milk
1 small banana, sliced
1 slice whole wheat toast, with
    1 teaspoon reduced-calorie soft margarine
4 ounces orange juice

LUNCH

1 tuna salad sandwich, made with
    3½ ounces canned water-packed tuna, drained
    ¼ cup chopped celery
    1 tablespoon chopped onion (optional)
    2 tablespoons mayonnaise
    ½ medium tomato, sliced
    ½ cup shredded lettuce
    1 medium pita bread
½ medium cucumber, cut into spears
1 medium apple
Beverage

DINNER

2 Broiled Lamb Chops (4 ounces total), lean only (see recipe)
½ cup cooked rice, with
    ½ teaspoon reduced-calorie soft margarine
1 cup cooked fresh or frozen peas and carrots, with
    1 teaspoon reduced-calorie soft margarine
2 cups tossed garden salad, with
    2 tablespoons reduced-calorie salad dressing
1 strawberry sundae, made with
    ½ cup vanilla ice milk
    1 cup fresh strawberries
1 cup acidophilus low-fat milk

SNACKS

2 cups popped popcorn
1 medium orange
1 peppermint milkshake (see Milkshake Marvel recipe)

DAY 7 **Wednesday**

BREAKFAST

2 pancakes, 4 inches in diameter, with
    1 teaspoon reduced-calorie soft margarine
½ cup fresh blueberries
4 ounces unsweetened pineapple juice
1 cup acidophilus low-fat milk

LUNCH

1 cheese sandwich, made with
    2 ounces Swiss cheese
    lettuce
    ½ teaspoon mustard
    2 slices rye bread
1 medium raw carrot, cut into sticks
1 celery stalk, cut into sticks
3 fresh medium apricots
Beverage

DINNER

4 ounces baked skinless chicken breast
½ cup stuffing
1 cup fresh summer squash, with
    1 teaspoon reduced-calorie soft margarine
½ cup lima beans, with
    ½ teaspoon reduced-calorie soft margarine
1 tablespoon cranberry sauce
2 cups tossed garden salad, with
    2 tablespoons reduced-calorie salad dressing
½ cup unsweetened applesauce
1 cup acidophilus low-fat milk

SNACKS

2 cups popped popcorn
1 large tangerine
1 Chocolate Milkshake (see recipe)

24

A SLIM NEW LIFE

Is the You Can Do It! Kids Diet really worth it? Is it worth all the time it takes? All the effort you must make? All the responsibility you must take? All the temptations you must endure? And the total commitment you must pledge? You bet it is!

In the weeks and months after you reach your goal, there is no doubt in your mind. Your life has changed for the better in so many ways. Food used to be numero uno when you were gaining weight. But now food plays a lesser role. You have finally learned that there is so much more to life than food. That means you are more active than ever before, doing things you only dreamed about doing. You have changed physically. Your body is lean and primed with energy. Your hair shines, your skin glows.

But the most important change is the one that takes place inside your head. Your dieting success has inspired you with a dynamic feeling of accomplishment that carries over into all facets of your life: at school, at home, at play, and in public. You have won! And just knowing that fact can give you the edge you need to reach whatever other goals you have set for yourself in life. You are brimming with a tremendous sense of self-confidence. No ribbon, no trophy, no certificate can mean as much to you as the knowledge that you have achieved a goal that once seemed impossible to reach. For the rest of your life, you can always remember that when faced with a difficult challenge you rose to the occasion. You mustered up the determination to succeed. You can rely on that strength now in whatever else you want to achieve, whether it's to make the honor roll, have new friends, learn to ski, become a model, win first place in the regional debate finals, or simply be a nicer person.

Is this diet really worth it? Ask any of the thousands of young people who have already lost weight on the You Can Do It! Kids Diet. They can tell you what a slim new life means to them. Read what some of the formerly overweight young people in my classes have to say:

Nick, twenty, lost 47 pounds and has been at his goal for five years: The best thing I ever did in my life was lose weight. In ninth grade I was 5 feet, 8 inches tall and weighed 204 pounds. I was so fat that I was exhausted from climbing stairs at school to get from my homeroom to science class. The doctor said I had high blood pressure and that I couldn't participate in P.E. because I was too out of shape. I was going nowhere. I didn't have any ambitions. I didn't have many friends and what friends I did have often poked fun at me. All my brothers were into sports and I finally wised up and decided I was missing out on too many things. I went on the diet and it changed my life. My blood pressure dropped to normal. I made the wrestling team and won thirty-eight matches and lost only nineteen. Girls started looking at me, whereas before it was only the other way around. I went to the beach every chance I got. I never did that when I was fat. To me, the diet helped in so many other ways. It taught me patience. Sometimes during wrestling season or football season when the going got tough, I'd tell myself, "I didn't go through all this dieting to give up." I applied that same determination to my everyday life. I don't give up. I'm in college now and I have some definite goals for my life and I intend to reach them. I'm happy about who I am and what I have accomplished.

Marianne, fifteen, lost 30 pounds and has been at her goal for two years: I feel reborn. Every day is wonderful. Now that I'm no longer fat, my whole life is so much happier. Let me put it to you this way: Guys, guys, and more guys! Clothes, clothes, and more clothes! My closet is bursting instead of the backside of my jeans.

Stephanie, sixteen, lost 65 pounds and has been at her goal one year: During my first year in high school I weighed 205 pounds. I didn't belong to anything other than the human race. Most of my free time was spent alone in my room just twirling a baton. I finally decided I wanted more out of my life, so I went on the diet. I can't describe what losing all that weight has meant to me. It's like I've been released from prison and I'm free to do whatever I want. I am a majorette in the high school marching band, I'm in the school chorus, and I'm a member of several other clubs on campus. I'm not ashamed of my body like I used to be and I feel proud of the changes I've made. What I like the best is when people ask me if I was "that fat girl." I tell them that was another life I had.

Joshua, fifteen, lost 42 pounds and has been at his goal for six months: I haven't changed that much on the inside. But now that I am no longer overweight, people give me a chance to show them who I really am and what I'm capable of doing.

Jillian, twelve, lost 33 pounds and has been at her goal for one year: I really like the new me. I can even say I'm great now. How about that? Me great, instead of great big me! I love being normal.

Patti, sixteen, lost 58 pounds and has been at her goal for three years: Now I'm doing great in school, I have a boyfriend, I work part-time in a boutique, and I've learned to scuba dive. All of these things came true because I made them come true. But they wouldn't have happened if I had stayed fat. I was miserable, depressed, and felt that anyone else on earth looked better than I did. I sure don't feel that way anymore. I take pride in my appearance. I make sure my makeup is just right, my hair is in place, and my clothes are spotless. I feel good about myself and I've seen how my personality has changed. I'm much more outgoing than before. Also, I'm more aware of people and their feelings and I think that explains why I seem to have many more friends. They didn't flock to me just because I lost all that weight. Because of my self-confidence, I went to them. I am so happy about what I've done.

Bob, fifteen, lost 40 pounds and has been at his goal for one year: Since hitting my goal, the two most important things in my life are football and girls. I couldn't say that last year. Back then I was a fat slob. It hurts to say that, but it was true. I didn't care if I had stains on my shirt or went without a belt or didn't comb my hair. I always tried to be nice to girls, but I knew they wouldn't have anything to do with me, so I never tried to ask them out or anything like that. Last year I was a second stringer on the football team as an offensive guard. I didn't play very much because I couldn't run very fast. All I did was huff and puff. The coach was always on my case about losing weight, but I wouldn't listen until I reached the point where I knew if I got much bigger, I'd explode. I went from a size 38 men's in pants to a size 32. Now I wear a belt because it accents my waist. I'm very conscious about my appearance and I take good care of my hair and complexion. I really like girls and for the first time in my life I'm discovering they like me. Man, let me tell you, I wish I had gone on a diet years ago. This year on the football team I'm starting linebacker, and I made two interceptions in the first two games of the season. I don't know if losing weight has anything to do with it, but during the first grading period this year I had the best grades since fifth grade. I know one thing. I never want to be fat again. I missed out on too many things. But never again. I honestly believe I can go out and do whatever I want to accomplish. That may sound conceited, but to me that's the truth.

Heidi, thirteen, lost 35 pounds and has been at her goal for nine months: When I started this diet, I always thought and dreamed that when I became thinner, I'd be the most popular kid in school and the star on the girls' soccer team. Well, that didn't happen. But I'm not disappointed because a lot of other good things have happened to me since I lost weight. I've finally realized that it's fun just to be me. Now I can concentrate on my grades and do things without being afraid. I never used to raise my hand in class because I was sure that if I gave the wrong answer, the rest of the class would laugh at me and then call me fat names. Now I talk a lot because I have something to say. When I was fat I didn't like myself but I knew that under all that fat was a pretty nice person. I like myself a whole lot more now. Physically, I run faster and I play better on the soccer team but I'll never be the star because I don't have the talent. Still, I enjoy playing, and the coach told me I have improved quite a bit so that makes me feel good. Before I lost weight I was scared of people because I knew that they would tease me. If anyone told a funny joke, I would never laugh because I was so ashamed about being fat that I didn't want anyone to know I was around. Now I think I have a pleasant personality and I enjoy being around other people. I never thought I'd feel this good about myself.

You owe it to yourself to give your body the very best care it deserves. So make up your mind to get started on this diet right now. It could be the greatest gift you've ever given yourself. I know one thing: YOU CAN DO IT!

Dear Parent . . .

Up to this point I have directed my remarks solely to your son or daughter. Now I want to turn my attention to you.

But first I am going to make two assumptions: (1) You have read the book so you understand what kind of food and responsibilities are involved in making this diet work. (2) Your child, for whom this book is intended, has read (or will read) this chapter.

I'm writing to you because I have found in my diet classes that there are many things young dieters want to make sure that their parents know.

As you are aware, I stress that each young person must take full responsibility for losing weight on this diet. But the truth is that without your support—in fact, without the support and cooperation of the whole family—your child will have an extremely difficult time reaching his goal. You can make the difference between his success or failure.

Showing support means much more than just an occasional pat on your child's back. It means making sure the right foods are always available, correcting the family's bad eating habits, cutting back on junk foods and big meals, showing patience and understanding, and giving encouragement.

Suzanne, fourteen, lost 25 pounds and was 9 pounds from her goal: It's nice to have parents who care. Sometimes Mom and Dad let me know they are proud of me and congratulate me when I've had a good week. That makes me feel good. I don't think I could've gone this far without their help.

Before your child begins the diet, let him explain to the whole family what losing weight means to him. Ask for suggestions from family members on how they can help, take a stand against teasing from brothers and sisters, and seek agreement on how to handle snacks and junk food in the house.

Because this diet makes no allowances for junk food and most canned, packaged, or convenience foods, it is very important that your child have the proper foods available at home. Otherwise there is no way in the world that he or she can lose the weight effectively.

Mother of Judy, eleven, who lost 13 pounds and was 10 pounds from her goal: Judy makes up her own list of foods that she needs for the week and I drive her to the store. It's fun for her to shop and it gives her a sense of responsibility and independence. I make sure that all the foods she needs are in the house. If I don't, the temptation is too great for her to grab whatever is on hand and make a dinner that she shouldn't be eating.

Encourage your child to take on as much responsibility as he can handle, from menu planning to grocery shopping, from making his lunches daily to weighing himself weekly. It's your child's diet, not yours.

Chances are your child is going to feel different if for no other reason than he is on a diet, so do your best to minimize this feeling when you gather around the table to eat. Make your child feel that he is still very much a part of the family at dinnertime. Don't make him feel like an outcast because the diet calls for a dinner completely different from what the rest of the family is eating.

While your child is coping with a whole new way of eating, you can help tremendously by making a few simple adjustments in your menu planning. Show your support by eating the same types of simple meals that he must now eat. It will lessen the chance of temptation and frustration. Besides, you benefit too, because the meals are delicious, filling, and nutritious. The only difference between his meals and yours is that you can eat larger amounts.

If preparing low-calorie meals for the whole family seems too unappealing to you, then at least try to build your dinners around what your child is eating—especially during the first two weeks when he is getting accustomed to a new way of eating. I discussed this suggestion in chapter 19, "Coping at Home," but it is so important that it bears repeating. You can make the same basic dinner, except that you can add sauces and gravies for the other members of your family.

Mother of Kim, fifteen, who lost 25 pounds and was 10 pounds from her goal: Usually our meals are not that much different from Kim's because I want the whole family to eat in a healthy way. But I don't deprive the other children of their favorite foods just because Kim is on a diet. We still have our spaghetti or macaroni and cheese or mashed potatoes and gravy. However, we did wait until she was a few weeks into the diet before we ate those kinds of things. I plan our heavy meals for the times when Kim is spending the night at a friend's house. Then we don't feel so guilty about what we eat.

Nobody says you must give up snacking. Just show a little compassion and understanding. It's pretty hard for your child not to notice if you devour a big bowl of ice cream while you watch TV. To avoid this situation, have your food treats when your child is elsewhere. It's a small price to pay for helping him lose weight, isn't it?

If you must have sweets and other snacks around the house, at least keep them out of sight so your child isn't constantly faced with temptation battles. Tell the other members of the family to eat their snacks and junk food only in the kitchen—not throughout the house—or outside.

Take an active interest in your child's dieting efforts. Show you care about his triumphs and troubles on the diet. Show you have confidence in him. Your failure to perform these simple acts could lead to his failure.

A few kind words that show you are behind him one hundred percent can give your child the boost he needs during difficult moments on the diet. But on the flip side of the coin, the wrong words can have a devastating effect. Sometimes we parents say things without realizing how damaging they can be to our children.

Mother of Debbie, fourteen, who lost 31 pounds and was 16 pounds from her goal: About halfway through her diet, I bought Debbie several new outfits because her old clothes were too loose. She put her old clothes in a box and said she wanted to give them away to the poor. Without thinking, I said, "Why don't we put those clothes back in your closet just in case . . ." I caught myself but not in time. She gave me a look that broke my heart and ran out of the room. I felt just awful. I let her down. Later, I apologized and told her that my remark was thoughtless and that I really did have complete confidence in her.

Father of Christie, thirteen, who lost 22 pounds and was 10 pounds from her goal: I did a real dumb thing. One day I was out in the yard talking to my neighbor about Christie's diet. In a light-hearted vein, I said, "So you know what her losing weight is doing to me? I'm going broke buying her new clothes." Christie overheard me and began to cry. I felt like two cents. She's sensitive about dieting. I should have known better.

How much or how little should a parent say to a child about the diet? That pretty much depends upon your relationship. Let your child lead the way in any conversations concerning the diet. Don't initiate the dialogue because it could seem as though you are nagging. One of the surest ways for a child to fall off the diet is to be nagged to death. You must give your child breathing room. If your child has read this book and understands this diet, there are strong indications that he has a high level of motivation for self-improvement. So all he or she needs from you is encouragement and perhaps some guidance.

If your child wants to talk about the diet, discuss it, but don't interrogate. And don't give lectures or sermons. That's a turnoff. Even if you have the greatest of intentions, it could backfire because it's difficult for a child to know the difference between a concerned parent and a nosy one. If he is making progress, you'll know it without having to ask. He will volunteer the information: "My belt goes over another notch." "Remember this dress that didn't fit before? Now it does."

Mother of Heidi, thirteen, who lost 35 pounds and reached her goal: I never asked Heidi her weight or how much she lost in any particular week. I never even brought up the subject of dieting. Only if she brought it up did we talk about it, and basically I would just listen to whatever she had to say. I'd ask her, "Did you have a good week?" or I'd compliment her on her progress or her looks. She wanted this diet to be her private thing, so I stepped out of the picture. I just made sure I had the food she needed in the house. I also made sure I was there when she did need me to listen.

Mother of Michael, sixteen, who lost 18 pounds and was 34 pounds from his goal: I stay out of his diet entirely, other than making sure he has the right kind of food available to him in the house. If I say anything about his diet, I usually end up making it worse, so we agreed it's best if I don't ask any questions unless he brings it up. I will give him a compliment every now and then on how good he's looking. I buy what he needs to eat but he fixes his own dinners. By doing all of these things, we get along better.

Sometimes your child may want to talk about food. This often defuses the issue of temptation and your child may be less likely to run to the store and buy something fattening. He might say, "I remember how delicious your strawberry pie was." This is not self-inflicted torture. Many young people need to talk it out, to relieve any built-up frustration. Better to talk about food than eat it.

What happens when you see your son or daughter trying to sneak a piece of cake? Do you come down hard on him for committing an "oops"? Unless your child is pretty young and needs to be told what to do, I suggest you look the other way. He is entitled to make a few mistakes during the diet. If your child is determined to lose weight, he will go right back on the diet. The less said from you about the oops the better. You don't want to make your child feel as though he is under constant surveillance, that you don't trust him. However, if you see a pattern developing of one oops after another, then perhaps you should approach your child in a calm manner and try to talk it out. If he can't handle the diet, then he is not ready to lose weight. But I can almost guarantee you that constant parental nagging will send even a dedicated dieter into an eating binge.

Mother of Helen, thirteen, who lost 8 pounds and was 10 pounds from her goal: I don't nag. Everyone makes mistakes. I've caught Helen eating something she shouldn't, but I don't say anything and she appreciates that. She is old enough to know that she made a mistake and the less said about it the better. She'll forget about it the next day and go back on her diet.

Mother of Kevin, twelve, who lost 17 pounds and was 7 pounds from his goal: Sometimes he gets discouraged. He starts complaining and saying he's tired of the diet and he asks for my advice. That's when I give him a pep talk: "It's your choice. You are doing a great job and I'd hate to see you give up all that you've worked for. We are very proud of you. Think how you are going to feel if you give up now. Remember what it was like before you went on the diet? You don't want to go back to that, do you?" He understands and I think he appreciates the concern.

This diet is not a punishment for overweight children. It is not a reason for parents to feel sorry for their fat kids. Parents who wrongly believe their little darlings are suffering when they diet usually make matters worse because they offer food treats. Such actions wreck all the good work that their dieting children have accomplished.

Father of Eric, twelve, lost 13 pounds and was 14 pounds from his goal: My son has stuck to the diet as best he can and I'm proud of his efforts. So every now and then I tell him to take a break from the diet and eat a dessert. His mother feels the same way I do. He deserves a treat.

Because of this ill-informed attitude, Eric's parents are not only prolonging his weight loss effort but also making it much more difficult for him to diet.

If you feel it's necessary to give your child an extra added incentive to lose weight, make it a nonfood reward such as a dollar per pound, or a trip to the ball park, or a weekend outing for every 10 pounds lost. Actually, the best rewards don't cost a penny. They are simple words of praise: "You really look good." "I am proud of the way you are handling the diet." "Keep it up, you look better than ever."

Some parents believe in offering a big reward if the

young person hits his goal. Such payoffs include weekend vacations, a new bicycle, or new clothes. In most cases, young people don't lose weight just so they can receive a prize. They lose weight because they want to improve their lives. They don't need other incentives.

Mother of Michelle, thirteen, who lost 44 pounds and reached her goal: We don't believe in giving rewards to Michelle. We wanted her to lose weight for herself. We also wanted to show her that the most important thing in life is knowing that you did something good for yourself. In the real world when you do something good for yourself nobody gives you presents. Throughout her diet, our role was to stand by her and offer her as much encouragement as possible. Our approach may not work for everybody but it sure worked for Michelle. Then again, she was highly motivated.

As your child loses weight, it's only natural that you are proud and want to brag about his success in much the same way you would if he achieved straight A's on a report card or hit the game-winning home run for the school team. But broadcasting his dieting success could put additional and unnecessary pressure on your child. Because dieting is often a sensitive subject to the young dieter, leave it up to him to tell others as much or little as he wishes about the diet.

Jake, fifteen, lost 38 pounds and reached his goal: When I lost about 30 pounds, my dad began telling everyone who walked through the door about how much weight I dropped. One day an insurance salesman came to call and my dad told him, "This is my son Jake. He's lost 38 pounds. What do you think of that?" Man, I wanted to hide from embarrassment. All I could do was force a smile and quickly excuse myself. That night I told my dad that I knew he was proud of me but from now on to please keep quiet and not tell the whole world how fat I was.

Diana, fifteen, lost 20 pounds and was 12 pounds from her goal: Mom embarrasses me sometimes. At the grocery store the other day, she told the checkout lady that I lost 20 pounds and Mom said, "Isn't that wonderful?" The lady nodded as if she really cared. I wondered what would've happened if the lady said "no." Then Mom told the lawn man that I am doing so good on my diet. I bet he thinks we are saving the grass clippings for my salads. I know Mom is thrilled to death for me, but this is ridiculous.

Please don't be put out by the suggestions I've made in this chapter. Certainly the few changes you may have to make are worth it. So little on your part can mean so much to your child. See for yourself. I asked parents to tell me how their children have changed as they lost weight. Here is a sampling of the parents' answers:

- ✔ "seems more assertive"
- ✔ "is much more self-confident"
- ✔ "has become involved in new activities"
- ✔ "is much more outgoing"
- ✔ "shows more patience"
- ✔ "seems calmer"
- ✔ "smiles again—all the time"
- ✔ "likes herself now"
- ✔ "dresses better"
- ✔ "loves the mirror"
- ✔ "talks with a positive attitude"
- ✔ "has lost the urge to be too critical about herself"
- ✔ "makes friends much more easily"
- ✔ "takes a greater interest in school"
- ✔ "is proud of her own accomplishments"
- ✔ "always seems in a good mood"
- ✔ "treats people with respect and kindness"

Father of Shelly, fourteen, who lost 14 pounds and reached her goal: Looking back, I feel a little guilty about not recognizing Shelly's weight problem earlier. Kids were calling her names and she was upset with her weight. She went on a diet by herself and we said, "Oh, that's nice," and that was the extent of our support. But she didn't stick with it very long. We began to worry that her poor self-image was causing her to eat more and more. One day she came to us and said she was tired of being fat. She said she was going on the You Can Do It! Diet and asked for our support. We told her we were with her all the way. We were very proud that she made the decision to try to lose weight and was doing this for herself. Our support meant more than words. It meant action. We based our meals around hers, got rid of all the junk food in the house, told the other kids in the house to respect Shelly's situation, and worked on improving our own eating habits. We agreed that if anyone wanted junk food, they'd have to eat it away from the house. I'm convinced that if we hadn't actively shown Shelly this kind of support, she never would have reached her goal. She is now an energetic, self-confident, beautiful girl. I'm very proud of her.

With your support throughout this diet, your child can do it. Your son or daughter will feel great—and so will you.

Some Other Books You'll Want to Read

EATING

Fretz, Sada. *Going Vegetarian: A Guide for Teenagers.* New York: Morrow, 1983.
Terrific reasons for turning to veggies, and lots of delicious and exotic recipes.

Huang, Paul C. *Illustrated Step-By-Step Beginner's Cookbook.* New York: Four Winds Press, 1980.
Detailed drawings break each recipe into easy stages for newcomers to the kitchen.

O'Neill, Cherry Boone. *Starving for Attention.* New York: Continuum, 1982. New York: Dell, 1983 (paper).
An explanation of anorexia nervosa and bulimia, two dangerous ways to overdo dieting.

Perl, Lila. *Junk Food, Fast Food, Health Food: What America Eats and Why.* Boston: Houghton-Mifflin, 1980.
How modern technology and big business have pushed our country into unhealthy eating.

EXERCISING

Columbu, Franco, and Dick Tyler. *Weight Training and Body Building: A Complete Guide for Young Athletes.* New York: Wanderer Books, 1979.

A champion weightlifter introduces young men to beginning, intermediate, and advanced techniques for working out with the heavy stuff.

Ferrigno, Lou, and Douglas Kent Hall. *The Incredible Lou Ferrigno*. New York: Simon and Schuster, 1981.
How the Incredible Hulk got to look that way.

Fonda, Jane. *Jane Fonda's Workout Book*. New York: Simon and Schuster, 1981.
The most popular exercise book ever.

Lyttle, Richard B. *The Complete Beginner's Guide to Physical Fitness*. New York: Doubleday, 1978.
Encouragement and lots of exercises for planning your own personal fitness routine.

Neale, Wendy. *On Your Toes: Beginning Ballet*. New York: Crown, 1980.
A get-ready book for new dancers, both girls and boys: how to choose a teacher, what to wear, and how to appreciate the performance world of professional ballet.

LOOKING GOOD

Bozic, Patricia. *The Sweet Dreams Fashion Book: Looking Hot Without Spending a Lot*. New York: Bantam, 1983 (paper).
A treasury of clever ideas for dressing inexpensively, but with dash.

Budd, Elaine. *You and Your Hair: Cuts, Styles, and Hints for Beautiful Hair*. New York: Scholastic (A Wildfire Book), 1978 (paper).
Understanding that stuff on top of your head and keeping it shiny and well styled.

McGrath, Judith. *Pretty Girl: A Guide to Looking Good, Naturally*. New York: Lothrop, 1981.
Beautiful photographs show how attractive healthy skin, hair, and a trim body can be. Good advice on young makeup and hair styles, too.

Zizmor, Jonathan, and Diane English. *Doctor Zizmor's Guide to Clearer Skin*. New York: Lippincott, 1980.
The causes of acne and good advice on ways to get rid of it.

SOME OTHER BOOKS YOU'LL WANT TO READ

FEELING HEALTHY

McCoy, Kathy. *The Teenage Body Book.* New York: Simon and Schuster, 1979 (paper).
Intelligent answers to teens' questions about medical, sexual, and health problems.

Simon, Nissa. *Don't Worry, You're Normal: A Teenager's Guide to Self-Health.* New York: Crowell, 1982 (also paper).
Up-to-date medical information on the physical changes and problems that are part of being a healthy teenager.

FEELING HAPPY

Booher, Dianna Daniels. *Making Friends with Yourself and Other Strangers.* New York: Julian Messner (Teen Survival Library), 1982.
Finding and keeping friends is a valuable skill that can be learned, but first you must shake your own hand.

Gilbert, Sara. *What Happens in Therapy.* New York: Lothrop, 1982.
How to find professional psychological help and what to expect from it.

Laiken, Deidre S., and Alan J. Schneider. *Listen to Me, I'm Angry.* New York: Lothrop, 1980.
Understanding and help for letting out anger in good ways.

McCoy, Kathy. *The Teenage Survival Guide: Coping with Problems in Everyday Life.* New York: Simon and Schuster, 1981 (paper).
Reassuring answers to teens' questions about parents, school, dating, love, friends, and other crises of growing up.

Vedral, Joyce L. *I Dare You: How to Use Psychology to Get What You Want out of Life: A Guide for Teenagers.* New York: Holt, Rinehart and Winston, 1983.
A simple and realistic technique for taking hold of your own life and making good things happen for you.

FICTION

Danziger, Paula. *The Cat Ate My Gym Suit*. New York: Delacorte, 1974. New York: Dell, 1975 (paper).
Overweight and insecure, thirteen-year-old Marcy Lewis comes out of her shell when she fights to save the job of a popular but controversial English teacher.

Greenberg, Jan. *The Pig-Out Blues*. New York: Farrar, Straus, 1982.
A neurotic, model-thin mother only complicates an overweight teenage daughter's problems with her life.

Holland, Isabelle. *Dinah and the Green Fat Kingdom*. New York: Lippincott, 1973. New York: Dell, 1981 (paper).
Dinah at twelve is a compulsive eater who takes refuge from her unhappiness in an imaginary Green Kingdom where everybody is fat.

Holland, Isabelle. *Heads You Win, Tails I Lose*. New York: Lippincott, 1973. New York: Dell, 1977 (paper).
Melissa gets thin enough to qualify for a part in the school play by gulping stolen diet and sleeping pills for weeks, but by try-out time she is too sick to care.

Kerr, M. E. *Dinky Hocker Shoots Smack!* New York: Harper, 1972. New York: Dell, 1973 (paper).
Dinky's anger at her family keeps her hiding under protective layers of fat, even when her self-confident (and overweight) boyfriend tries to get her to express the person she really is.

Knudson, R. R. *Zanboomer*. New York: Harper, 1978. New York: Dell, 1980 (paper).
A baseball injury forces Zan Hagen to turn her passion for excellence to a new sport—running.

Levenkron, Steven. *The Best Little Girl in the World*. Chicago: Contemporary Books, 1978. New York: Warner, 1983 (paper).
The terrifying secret life of a victim of anorexia nervosa, by a doctor who specializes in this disorder.

Lipsyte, Robert. *One Fat Summer*. New York: Harper, 1977. New York: Bantam, 1978 (paper).
Bobby Marks is sick and tired of being bullied and teased

about his weight, so he tackles a summer of lawn-cutting and diet, with hilarious but successful results.

Mazer, Harry. *The Island Keeper: A Tale of Courage and Survival.* New York: Delacorte, 1981. New York: Dell, 1982 (paper).

A rich but lonely fat girl survives on a remote Canadian island by her wits and her own two hands, to emerge a year later trim, strong, and confident.

Sachs, Marilyn. *The Fat Girl.* New York: Dutton, 1984.

Jeff's loathing for blubbery Ellen changes to an unhealthy fascination when he finds that he can control her—up to a point.

Shreve, Susan. *The Revolution of Mary Leary.* New York: Knopf, 1982. New York: Avon, 1984 (paper).

The only way Mary can get her life and her weight under her own control is to run away from her cookie-pushing mother's Serious Discussions.

Index

Acidophilus milk, 78, 210
Adults:
   likelihood of fat children becoming fat, 28
   problems of overweight, 27–28
   see also Family
Advertising, food, 30
Airplanes, eating on, 177
Amusement parks, eating at, 177–78
Anger:
   eating out of, 155, 195–96
   venting your, 155–56
Anorexia nervosa, 206–207
Appearance, sharpening your, 64, 134, 152–53
Appetite, 46
   the first two weeks, 130–31
   stop eating when you're full, 125–26
   see also Hunger
Apple slices, cinnamon, 118
Artificial sweetener, 79, 212
Ascorbic acid, see Vitamin C
Athletics, problems with, 8–9
   see also Physical activity
Attitudes toward food, 42–43
Author's battle with fat, 7–18

Baking food, 210
Balanced diet, 39–40
Banana chips, frozen, 119
Bawling yourself out for the last time, 63–64
Beans, dried, 37, 39
Beef, see Meat
Beverages, 210, 211
   choices of, on the Diet, 72–73
   drinking 32 ounces each day in addition to milk, 79
   with meals, limiting, 126
   sipping, 124
   see also Milk; Soft drinks; Water
Big-boned, being, 29–30
Binging, 195–96, 197
Birthday parties, 169–70
Blaming others for an oops!, 197–98
Blender, 105
Body measurements, 62–63, 65
Boiling food, 76, 210
Books to read, other, 241–45
Braising food, 76, 210
Bread, 38, 40
   for breakfast, on the Diet, 68
   French toast, whole wheat, 108–109

247

Bread (cont'd)
    for lunch or dinner, on the Diet, 72, 78
    pita, 72, 78, 113
Breakfast, 75
    fourteen-day sample menu, 81–97
    main choices for, on the Diet, 68
    recipes, 108–109
    seven-day sample maintenance menu, 218–24
    skipping, 45
Broiling food, 76, 210
Brothers, see Family
Burger Romano, 114
Butter, 38

Calcium, 39
Calories:
    burned in physical activity, 65
    daily suggested consumption of, 32
    eating too many, and gaining weight, 32–36
    "empty," 40
    to maintain ideal weight, 212–13
    nutrients supplying your, 40
    in sample seven-day maintenance menu, 212
    on the You Can Do It! Kids Diet, 2
Camp, coping at summer, 178–81
Candy, 158–59, 162, 164–65
Carbohydrates, 37–38
Carrot(s):
    cottage cheese salad, 110
    roast chicken-in-a-pan dinner, 114
    vegetable salad and dip, 110
    zucchini and, 117
Cereals, 38, 39
    choices of, on the Diet, 68, 75
    presweetened breakfast, 4
Charcoal-grilling food, 76, 166, 210
Cheating, 194–98
Cheddar cheese dip, vegetable-, 113
Cheese, 37, 39
    choices of, on the Diet, 70
    limit of number of portions of, each week, 70, 76
    pita bread, and mushroom pizza, 113
    vegetable-, dip, 113
Chicken, roast, -in-a-pan dinner, 114
    see also Poultry
Chocolate:
    milkshake, 122
    turtles, 117
Christmas season, 160–65
Cinnamon:
    apple slices, 118
    -margarine French toast topping, 109
Citrus fruits, 38
Cleaning your plate, 125
Clothes, 13, 15, 20, 64, 137–38
    buying, 11, 14–15, 24, 138, 233–34
    in goal size, 64, 303
Coffee, decaffeinated, 79
    milkshake, 120–21
College, 28
Comfort taken in food, 12, 42–43, 155
Commitment to lose weight, making a, 49–54
Compliments on weight loss, 15–16
Cooking methods, approved, 76, 80, 210
    ordering in restaurants, 172–73
    preparing meals and, 104–106
Coping on the Diet, 140, 143–98
Cornish hen, 111
Consignment shops, 138
Cottage cheese, 39
    salad, 110
    vegetable salad and dip, 110
Cucumber:
    cottage cheese salad, 110
    and tomato salad, 109

INDEX 249

Dairy products, 39, 211
  see also specific dairy products, e.g.
    Eggs; Milk; Yogurt
Dancing, 65
Dating, 10–11, 16, 26–27, 203, 205
Depression, 155
Desserts, 174
  chocolate turtles, 117
  cinnamon-apple slices, 118
  frozen banana chips, 119
  frozen grapes, 118
  fruity yogurt, 118–19
  recipes, 117–19
Diabetes, 28
Diary, *see* Personal journal
Diet, the, *see* You Can Do It! Kids Diet
Diet Encounter, 18
Dieting, failed attempts at, 12
Difficult weeks during the Diet, 137
Dining room, eating only in the kitchen or, 125
Dinner:
  fourteen-day sample menu, 81–97
  main choices for, on the Diet, 69–74
  seven-day sample maintenance menu, 218–24
Dip:
  vegetable-cheese, 113
  vegetable salad and, 110
Divorce, 189–91
Doctor(s), 13, 17
  consulting, before starting the Diet, 55
  setting weight goal with your, 61, 215
Dressings, *see* Salad dressing
Dried beans, 37, 39
Drinks, *see* Beverages

Ease-Up Day, 160–65, 169–70
Eating habits, 123–27
  bad, 41–45, 123

Eating Habits Quiz, 43–44
  family, 30–31, 183–85
  good, 123–27, 211
Eating Habits Quiz, 43–44
Eating slowly, 123–25
Eating the wrong food, 36–41
Eating the wrong way, 41–44
Eating too fast, 45–46
Eating too much, 32–36
Eggs, 39
  for breakfast, 68
  limit on number to eat each week, 68, 75–76
  pepper and onion scramble, 108
  whole wheat French toast, 108–109
Energy level, 137, 215
Equal, 79, 212
Excuses for being fat, 29–32
Exercise, *see* Physical activity

Family, 182–93
  advice for parents, 230–39
  bragging about child's weight loss, 237–38
  changes to expect from dieter, 238
  conflict at home, 23–24
  divorced parents who don't support the diet, 189–91
  eating big meals in front of you, 183–84, 232
  eating habits, 30–31, 183–85
  grandparents and relatives who ignore the diet, 191–93
  groceries for your diet and, 102–103, 231
  heredity and overweight, 30–31
  holding a meeting with your, 65–66, 231
  lack of encouragement from, 186–87
  nagging by, 187–88, 234
  snacking on junk food, 184–85, 232–33

Family (cont'd)
  support from, 13, 144, 182, 186–87, 193, 230–39
  teasing and tempting by, 11–12, 19–20, 23, 185–86, 231
  using food as reward, 188–89, 236
Family style, stop serving, 126
Farina, 39
Fast food restaurants, 171, 176–77
  temptation of, 149–50
Fat, 2–3
  the author's battle with, 7–18
  discrimination against the, 27–28
  problems of being, 19–28
  reasons you are, 29–46
Fats, dietary, 38, 40
  choice of, on the Diet, 74
  limiting your use of, 74, 80, 211
  on maintenance plan, 210
Fattening food, 40
  on Ease-Up Day, 161
  temptation of, 30
Fiber, 39–40, 77, 210
First two weeks on the Diet, 128–35
  gorging before, 128–29
  side effects to expect, 128–32
Fish, 37, 39, 210
  broiled, fillet, 112–13
  choices of, on the Diet, 69–70
Food shopping, 100–102, 231
Fourteen-day sample menu, 81–97
  getting enough to eat, 96
  plain foods on, 96–97
  starting on a Thursday, 96
Freezing individual portions, 106
French toast:
  topping, cinnamon-margarine, 109
  whole wheat, 108–109
Friends, 9–10, 26–27, 205
  talking about your feelings to, 148, 156–57
  temptation from, 147, 149–50, 156, 157

Fruit juices:
  choices of, on the Diet, 72
  substituting, for one of the fruit portions, 72, 78
Fruits, 38, 39
  choices of, on the Diet, 71–72
  eating three portions of fresh, daily, 77–78
  fruity milkshake, 121
  on maintenance plan, 209
  see also individual fruits
Fruity milkshake, 121
Fruity yogurt, 118–19
Frustration, eating out of, 155
Frying pan, nonstick, 76, 105, 106

Glandular problem, 29, 55
Goals:
  clothing size, 64, 203
  weight, 56–61, 136, 140, 201–207
Grains, 39–40, 210
Grandparents, 191–93
Grape-Nuts cereal, 118
  frozen banana chips, 119
Grapes, frozen, 118
Gravies, 210
Green pepper:
  burger Romano, 114
  cottage cheese salad, 110
  and onion scramble, 108
  and red pepper combo, 116
Grits, 40
Grocery shopping, 100–102, 231
Guidelines for the Diet, 74–80
  artificial sweeteners, 79
  cheese, limits on, 76
  cooking methods, approved, 76
  diet pills and appetite suppressants, do not buy, 80
  dietetic food, 80
  drinking at least 32 ounces of liquid daily, in addition to milk, 79

INDEX **251**

Guidelines for the Diet (*cont'd*)
   drinking three 8-ounce glasses of low-fat milk daily, 78
   eating salads, 77
   eating the right cereals, 75
   eating three complete meals a day, 75
   eating three portions of fresh fruit daily, 77–78
   eating 3 to 4 cups of vegetables daily, 76–77
   eggs, limits on number of, 75–76
   fats, limits on use of, 80
   meat, limits on high-fat, 76
   pita bread, 78
   seasoning your food, 79
   snacks, 80
   weighing and measuring food, 74
Guilt, 132, 155, 162, 195, 198
Gym class, 8–9, 22–23

Hair, 64, 134, 152
Halloween, 164–65
Headaches, 128, 129, 130, 134–35, 162
Health, dangers of overweight, 28
Heart attack, 28
Hen, Cornish, 111
   see also Poultry
Heredity, 30–31
High blood pressure, 28
Holidays and special events, coping on, 160–70
Home, coping at, *see* Family
Humor, sense of, 152
Hunger, 45–46, 96, 139
   the first two weeks, 130–31
   snacks only when you're hungry, 126
   stop eating when you're full, 125–26
   see also Appetite

Ice cream, 39
Ice crusher, 105
Ice milk, 39
Imagination:
   to resist temptation, 144–45
   visualizing yourself thin, 52, 55–56
Interviews, 28
Iron, 39

Jealousy, 132
Job interviews, 28
Journal, *see* Personal journal
Junk food, 127, 149–50, 162, 184–85, 211, 231, 232–33
"Just one" syndrome, 147

Kale, 39
Ketchup, 41
Kitchen, eating only in the dining room or, 125

Lamb chop, broiled, 111–12
Latchkey students, 148–49
Laxatives, 197
Lentils, 37
Letters to yourself, 62
Liquids, *see* Beverages
Liver, 38, 39
Low profile about your diet, keeping a, 151–52
Lunch:
   fourteen-day sample menu, 81–97
   main choices for, on the Diet, 69–74
   at school, 157–58
   seven-day sample maintenance menu, 218–24
Luncheon meats, 41

Main choices on the Diet:
   for breakfast, 68
   for lunch or dinner, 69–74
Main dish recipes, 111–15

252 INDEX

Maintaining your ideal weight, 16–17, 32, 207–24
  adjusting your ideal weight as you grow, 213–15
  determining how much to eat, 212–13
  fitness program, 215–16
  how to eat, 210–11
  increasing portion size, 209, 211
  as lifetime responsibility, 207, 208
  seven-day sample maintenance menu, 212, 217–24
  what to avoid, 211–12
  what to eat, 209–10
Margarine, 38, 74, 80
  cinnamon-, French toast topping, 109
Matthews, Dee (author):
  battle with fat, 7–18
  founding of program for the overweight, 18
Mayonnaise, 74
Meals:
  being presented with big, 31
  guidelines for the Diet, 74–80
  limiting beverages with, 126
  preparing, 104–106
  skipping, 45, 75
  taking time eating, 123–25
  what you can eat on the Diet, 68–74
  see also Breakfast; Dinner; Lunch; Menus
Measurements, *see* Body measurements
Measurements and weights, table of, 74
Measuring cups and spoons, 74
Measuring food, 74, 104
Meat, 37, 38, 39, 210
  burger Romano, 113–14
  buying lean, 106
  choices of, on the Diet, 69
  lamb chop, broiled, 111–12
  limit on number of portions of high-fat, each week, 69, 76
Menstrual period, 139
Menus:
  creating your own, 98–100
  family, 232
  fourteen-day sample, 81–97
  seven-day sample maintenance, 212, 217–24
Microwave oven, cooking in a, 76, 106
Milk, 37, 38, 39
  acidophilus, 78, 210
  allergy, 78
  on the Diet, 73
  drinking three 8-ounce glasses of low-fat, daily, 78
  milkshakes, 120–22
Milkshakes, 120–22
  chocolate, 122
  coffee, 120–21
  fruity, 121
  marvel, 121–22
  piña colada, 120
  sunshine orange, 122
Mineral supplements, 55
Mineral water, 79
Moodiness, 131–33
Mozzarella cheese, pita bread and mushroom pizza, 113
Mushroom(s):
  pita bread cheese and, pizza, 113
  seasoned, 115
Mustard, 39, 41

Nagging by parents, 187–88, 234
  about an oops!, 235
Negative self-image, 25–26
Niacin, 38, 39
Notebook, *see* Personal journal

NutraSweet, 79, 212
Nutrients, 37–40, 209
Nuts, 37, 38, 39

Oatmeal, 38
Oils, 38
Olives, 41
Onion:
   burger Romano, 114–15
   pepper and, scramble, 108
Oops!, handling an, 194–98
   what parents should do, 235–36
Orange juice, sunshine orange milkshake, 122
Overeating, see Eating too much

Parents, see Family
Parties, coping at, 166–70
Pasta, 38, 40
Patience, lack of, 131–32
Peas, 37
Pep talk, giving yourself a, 137
Pepper:
   burger Romano, 114–15
   cottage cheese salad, 110
   green and red, combo, 116
   and onion scramble, 108
Personal journal, 61–63
Personality, 205–206
Photographs of yourself, 62
   to help you cope with temptation, 146, 147
Physical activity, 181, 196, 203, 205, 213
   athletics, 8–9
   becoming more active, 64–65
   calorie needs and, 32
   during the holidays, 162, 165
   gym class, 8–9, 22–23
   as part of maintenance plan, 215–16

Physican, see Doctor(s)
Pickles, 41
Picnics, holiday, 165
Pineapple:
   chocolate turtles, 117
   piña colada milkshake, 120
Pita bread, 72, 78
   cheese and mushroom pizza, 113
Plain foods, 96–97
Planning ahead for weekly menus, 102–103
Plateaus in weight loss, 138–39
Popcorn, 74, 80
Pork, 38
Positive thinking, 132, 134, 153, 198
Posture, 64, 152
Potato:
   on the Diet, 71, 77
   roast chicken-in-a-pan dinner, 114
Potato chips, 41, 211
Poultry, 37, 38, 39, 210
   see also Chicken; Cornish hen
Premenstrual water retention, 139
Preparations for starting the Diet, 55–66
   bawl yourself out, 63–64
   buy an outfit in your goal size, 64
   get a good scale, 63
   get physical, 64–65
   hold a family meeting, 65–66
   set a target date, 61
   set a weight goal, 56–61
   sharpen your appearance, 64
   start a personal journal, 61–62
   take body measurements, 62–63
   take photographs of yourself, 62
   visit your doctor, 55
   write letters to yourself, 62
Preparing meals, 104–106
   don't sample food while, 127
Pretzels, 41
Protein, 37, 39, 40, 210

254 INDEX

Public, problems of overweight kids in, 24–25
Public Health Bulletin, 30

Quiz, Eating Habits, 43–44

Recipes, 107–22
   breakfast, 108–109
   consulting the index for, 82
   dessert, 117–19
   main dish, 111–15
   milkshakes, 120–22
   salad, 109–10
   vegetable side dishes, 115–17
Red pepper and green pepper combo, 116
Relatives, *see* Family
Responsibility for your weight, 31–32, 49–52, 153–54, 230
   reaching your weight goal, 140, 201–207
   a slim new life, 225–29
Restaurant style, serving, 126
Restaurants:
   coping in, 171–74, 177
   fast-food, 149–50, 171, 176–77
Retinol, *see* Vitamin A
Reward(s), 101
   food as a, 42, 188–89, 236
   nonfood, 126–27, 136, 189, 236–37
Riboflavin, *see* Vitamin B2
Roasting food, 76

Salad bars, 173
Salad dressing, 38, 106, 173
   on the Diet, 74, 77
Salads, 106
   cottage cheese, 110
   on the Diet, 77
   recipes, 109–10
   tomato and cucumber, 109
   vegetable, and dip, 110
   see also Vegetables
Salt, *see* Sodium
Sampling food while cooking, 127
Sardines, 39
Sauces, 210
Sausage, 41
Scale:
   for weighing food, 74, 104
   for weighing yourself, 63
School:
   coping in, 151–59
   grades, 9–10
   lunch at, 157–58
   participating in activities at, 152, 158–59
   problems of overweight kids at, 22–23, 151–52
Seafood, 210
   choices of, on the Diet, 60–70
   skewered shrimp, 112
Seasoned mushrooms, 115
Seasonings on the Diet, 73, 79
Second helpings, 126
Self-confidence, 16
   lack of, 9, 13, 20–21, 25–26
   a slim new life, 225–29
Seltzer, 79
Sense of humor, 152
Serving of meals, 126, 133
Shopping list, 100–101, 231
Shortening, 38
Shrimp, skewered, 112
Siblings, *see* Family
Sick, eating when you're, 137
SilverStone pans, 76, 106
Sipping beverages, 124
Sisters, *see* Family
Skin care, 64, 134
Skipping meals, 45, 75, 139
Slim new life, 225–29
Slumber parties, 168
Snacks, 74, 211, 232–33
   only when you're hungry, 232–33

Social activities, 16, 158, 203, 205–206
 dating, 10–11, 26–27, 203, 205
 missing, 9–11, 13, 20, 26–27
Soda, *see* Soft drinks
Sodium, 41, 79, 212
Soft drinks, 41, 79, 211
Special events and holidays, coping on, 160–65
Spices on the Diet, 73
Sports, *see* Physical activity
Spray-on vegetable coating for cooking, 80
Steamer, 105
Steaming food, 76, 77, 210
Stewing food, 76
Stomachaches, 128, 129, 130, 134–35, 162
Storage tips, 106
Strawberries, fruity yogurt, 118–19
Stroke, 28
Success rate of Diet, 3
Success stories, 226–29
Sugar, 40–41, 211–12
Summer camp, coping at, 178–80
Support:
 from family, 13, 144, 182, 186–87, 193, 230–39
 from friends, 148
Sweeteners, 212
 on the Diet, 73, 79
Sweets, avoiding, 211–12
Swimming, 65
Swiss Miss mix:
 chocolate milkshake, 122
 chocolate turtles, 117
 frozen banana chips, 119

Talking about your feelings, 148, 198, 234, 235
Target date for reaching your weight goal, 61
Tea, 79
Teasing about being fat or being on a diet, 8–9, 11–12, 19–20, 22–27, 151–55, 157, 159, 185–86, 231
Temper, short, 131–32
Temptation, coping with, 101, 140, 143–50
 see also Coping on the Diet
Thanksgiving-to-New Year's holiday season, 160–65
Tiredness, 130
Thiamin, *see* Vitamin B1
Thyroid gland, 29, 55
Tomato:
 burger Romano, 114–15
 and cucumber salad, 109
 Italiano, broiled, 116
 pita bread cheese and mushroom pizza, 113
Tooth decay, 211
Turnip greens, 39

Vacations, coping on, 175–81
Vegetables, 38, 39, 79, 106, 210
 -cheese dip, 113
 choices of, on the Diet, 70–71
 cooking methods for, 77
 eating 3 to 4 cups of, daily, 76–77
 on maintenance plan, 209
 recipes for side dishes, 115–17
 salad and dip, 110
 see also Salads; *individual vegetables*
Visualizing yourself thin, 52, 55–56
Vitamin A, 38, 39
Vitamin B1 (Thiamin), 38, 39
Vitamin B2 (Riboflavin), 38, 39
Vitamin C, 38, 39
Vitamin supplements, 55

Walking, 65
Water, 41, 79, 210
 retention of, 41, 139

Weekly menus:
  creating your own, 98–100
  planning ahead for, 102–103
  sample, 81–97, 217–24
Weighing food, 74, 104
Weighing yourself, 63, 134, 135
  during maintenance plan, 212–13
Weight charts, 57–60
  how to use, 57–61, 213–15
Weight gain, 197, 213
  adjusting your ideal weight as you grow, 213–15
Weight goal:
  knowing when to stop losing weight, 206–207
  plateau, 138–39
  reaching your, 140, 201–207
  setting a, 56–61
  short-term goals, 136
  target date for reaching your, 61
  see also Maintaining your ideal weight
Weight loss:
  anorexia nervosa, 206–207
  expected, 2, 133–34, 139
  the last few pounds, 139–40
  plateaus, 138–39
  the week of an oops!, 196–97
Weight reduction camps, 179–80
Weights and measurements, table of, 74
Wok, 76, 77, 210
Wrong food, eating the, 36–41

Yogurt, 38, 39
  on the Diet, 73, 78
  fruity, 118–19
You Can Do It! Kids Diet, 1–3, 67–68
  advice for parents, 230–39

coping at home, 182–93
coping at parties, 166–70
coping in restaurants, 171–74
coping in school, 151–59
coping on holidays and at special events, 160–65
coping on vacations and summer camp, 175–81
coping with temptation, 140, 143–50
creating menus of your own, 98–100
daily calorie consumption on, 2
day of the week to start, 96
the first two weeks, 128–35
fourteen-day sample menu, 81–97
grocery shopping, 100–102, 231
guidelines for the, 74–80
maintaining your ideal weight, 207–24
making up your mind, 49–54
"oops," handling an, 194–98
planning ahead, 102–103
preparations for going on the, 55–66
preparing meals, 104–106
reaching your goal, 140, 201–207
recipes, 82, 107–22
the rest of the way, 136–40
seven-day sample maintenance menu, 212, 217–24
a slim new life, 225–29
success rate of, 3
weight loss on, expected, 2, 133–34, 139
what you can eat, 68–74

Zucchini and carrots, 117